Dr. Mary has done an exceptional job distilling the science of lifestyle medicine into actionable nuggets of good health. Her approach to good health is a sure-fire way to achieve your best health starting today. Fingers, feet and forks are the "secret" to good health, and Dr. Mary teaches you how to use all three to move from surviving to thriving.

—STEPHAN ESSER, MD, FOUNDER OF ESSER HEALTH

I have placed **Waist Away** on my required reading list for my friends, private patients and family members; all the people who matter the most to me. Please feel free to listen to the interview at www.bullheadurgentcare.com and read Dr. Mary's book so that you too will no longer fail.

—DON WAGNER, DO, MEDICAL DIRECTOR OF BULLHEAD URGENT CARE AND HOST OF THE DR. DON SHOW

Waist Away was wasting away on my book shelf for a few months. I had no idea what I was missing! I love this book! Recipes, true stories of real people getting healthy and learning compassion, interviews with some of my favorite visionaries for compassionate living. I cannot figure out how all these treasures got stuffed into this small book! Thanks for creating this Mary and Chelsea!

—RAE SIKORA, NON-VIOLENCE/COMPASSIONATE LIVING ADVOCATE AND EDUCATOR

MARY CLIFTON, MD AND CHELSEA M CLINTON, MD

Waist Away

HOW TO JOYFULLY LOSE WEIGHT
AND SUPERCHARGE YOUR LIFE

FOREWORD BY NEAL D BARNARD, MD   INTRODUCTION BY MICHAEL GREGER, MD

Yes, we're doctors. But we're not your doctors. In medical studies and in our own private practices, people who change to a healthy, plant-based diet often require modifications to their medicines after they decrease their cholesterol or blood pressure. Changes often happen in just a few short weeks. Required insulin doses decrease dramatically, almost immediately after changing your diet. If you're not paying attention, you could experience low blood sugar reactions if you currently administer insulin. Be sure that you modify your diet under the supervision of your doctor.

We know what you're thinking. Potato chips are vegan. You're right, but they're also loaded with unhealthy fats and acrylamides, which are chemicals that concentrate in fried foods. Eating vegan junk food will just make you a fat and unhealthy vegan, not a goddess. We promote a whole-foods, plant-based diet to support your nutrition perfectly. Don't substitute a fried chip where a whole baked potato should be. We truly hope you will find the good health and joyful life that this healthy diet will bring you.

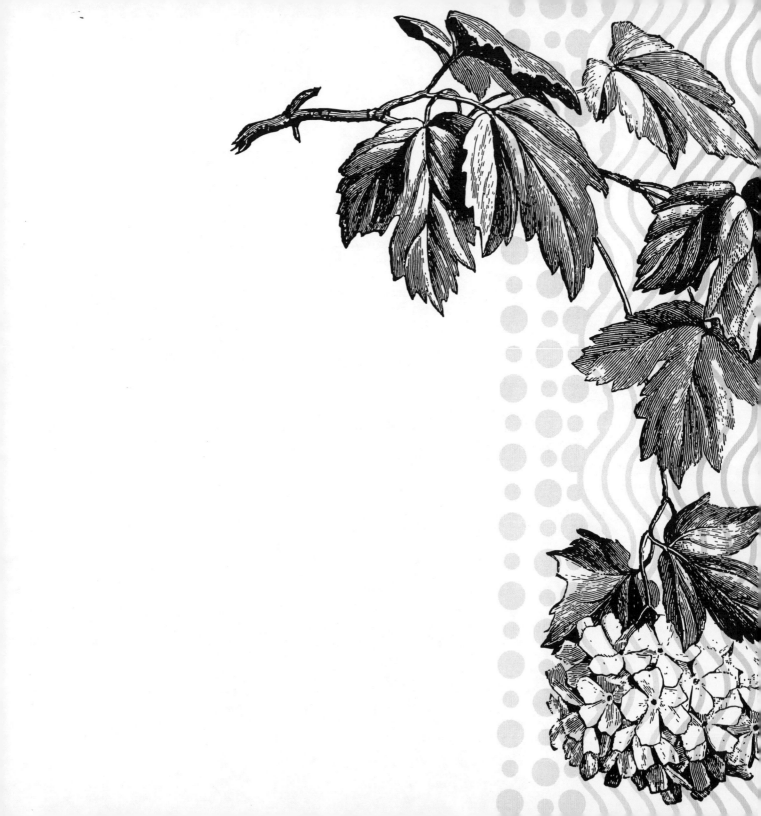

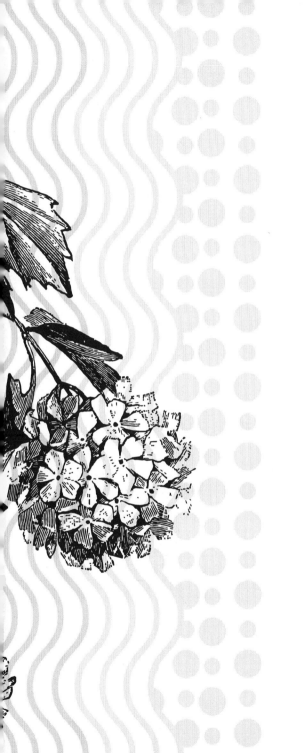

Contents

Recipes

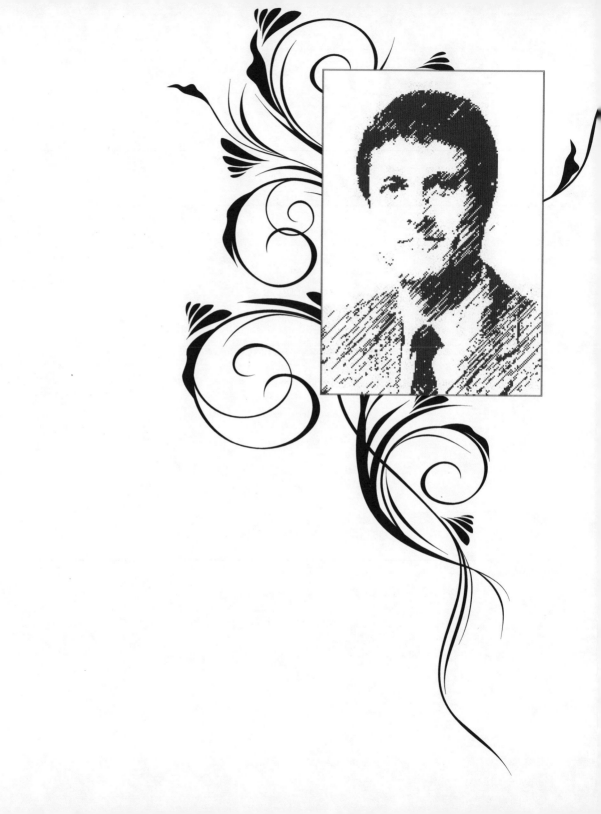

Waist Away will change your life. So many of us would like to eat better, slim down, and get healthy. But how do we go about it? So many diets turn out to be false starts. Sometimes they leave us worse off than when we began, and we wonder if we'll ever succeed. Well, set all that aside. You now have exactly the guide you need.

Mary Clifton, MD, and Chelsea Clinton, MD, are experts. In their clinical work, they have seen so many people whose weight problems or health problems seemed insurmountable. Between the two of them, they have seen it all. And they know how to help. In this book, they will bring you exactly the guidance you need.

The key is not to try to starve yourself thin, or to be miserly with carbs. Rather, the answer is to rethink the foods you are eating and to focus on those that deliver real health power. It is simple, and you will be surprised at how powerful it can be. This book will help you set aside the myths and get on the path to success.

In our research studies at the Physicians Committee for Responsible Medicine in Washington, DC, we have seen how simple changes to the menu can help people tackle an overly active appetite, boost a sluggish metabolism, and slim down once and for all. And more than that, they can help you improve and sometimes even reverse serious health conditions.

This book is a practical guide that will get you onto the right path, answer your questions, and hold your hand along the way. You'll see.

It really will change your life.

Neal D. Barnard, MD

President, Physicians Committee for Responsible Medicine

Washington, DC

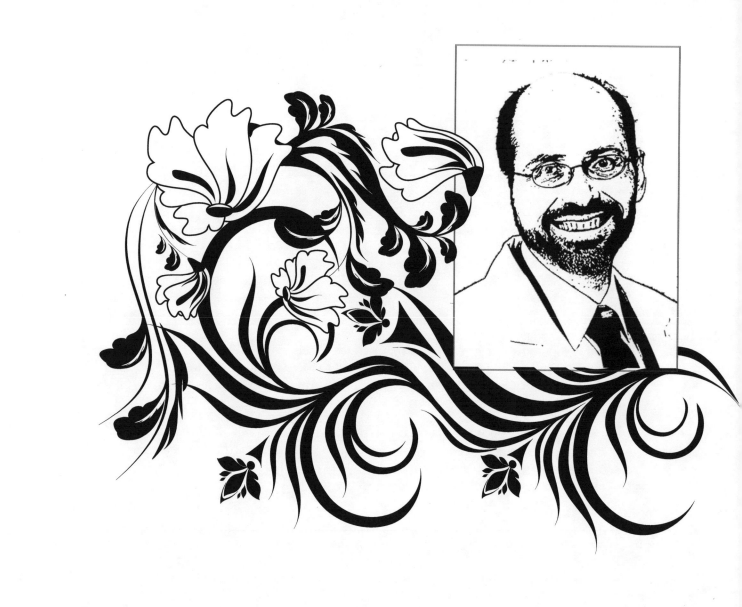

Every year, we North Americans spend more than $50 billion on diet products and self-help books and videos. It appears, however, that much of that money is being wasted. Western society continues to suffer an alarming epidemic of obesity and other "diseases of affluence" such as Type II diabetes, coronary heart disease and certain forms of cancer.

I believe that a significant part of the problem is that individuals—looking for guidance on the best diet to choose—are faced with a deluge of confusing and conflicting nutritional advice. My goal is to clarify the overwhelming "wealth" of information. Each year, I scour scientific journals for health-related studies for the latest in nutrition and health research. I interpret the data into plain English and present the findings on my website, nutritionfacts.org.

Much of what I've found in these thousands of studies each year points to a consistent conclusion. Eating a plant-based diet—one with no animal proteins—is the best possible thing you can do for your health, your weight, and your sense of well-being. Study after study delivers the general conclusion that it's better to get your medicine from vegetables and fruits than a pill bottle—or sadly, in the case of the chronically ill, a dozen or more pill bottles. As Hippocrates so wisely said thousands of years ago: "Our food shall be our medicine. Our medicine should be our food."

Dr. Mary Clifton has emerged with a strong and lively voice, advocating for just what all this research is showing. Americans who eat a plant-based diet are skinnier and healthier, on average, than those who eat meat. She is a researcher, but also, importantly, a physician. She works with patients who struggle with weight and chronic disease. Like most folks in this country, her patients know that diet and exercise will go a long way toward solving their problems. But knowing and acting are two different things. As a committed vegan herself, Dr. Mary walks the talk. She shows her patients how fundamental changes in their diet can completely transform their health, just as it did her own. Education has become her weapon of choice. And now she is publishing this book to spread the word further. Eating plants is not only good for your waistline, it's also good for your heart, your liver, your kidneys and your brain, not to mention the billions of animals that are killed each year to fill up America's dinner plates.

If you come to the table as a skeptic, you are not alone. Americans are deluged by conflicting results and news stories. But as a physician dedicated to sorting out the facts, I am here to say the evidence is consistent and mounting: vegans and vegetarians are statistically skinnier and healthier—and they suffer a much lower incidence of coronary heart disease, high blood pressure, certain types of cancer, gall stone and large intestine disorders. It's not only how long you live. It's also about how you live in your later years—in a doctor's office or playing on the tennis court?

For decades, only very small populations of vegans were involved in clinical studies. But that changed in 2009 when results of a study of thousands of U.S. vegans were published in the Journal of the American Diabetes Association.

In essence, researchers of the Loma Linda University School of Public Health compared what people ate and how much they weighed by measuring the body mass index (BMI) of each subject. A BMI over 30 is considered obese; between 25 and 30 is overweight. A BMI under 25 used to be considered "normal," but it's no longer the norm—not even close to the norm. According to the Centers for Disease Control and Prevention, nearly three out of four adult Americans are overweight or obese.

So let's look at the study and its conclusions on how diet affects weight. The average BMI of omnivores in the study was 28.8. Flexitarians weighed in at a BMI of 27.3 (a flexitarian is a flexible vegetarian who, in the study, is defined as someone who eats meat once or twice a month). Pesco-vegetarians, defined as vegetarians who eat fish, were overweight, too, with a bit lower BMI of 26.3. And what about vegetarians, who completely cut out meat? Well, this is America with all its temptations, and even the vegetarians were overweight with a 25.7 BMI. But they were at a significantly healthier weight than those who eat meat, even the flexitarians who reported eating meat only two to three times a month.

You can see where this trend is going.

What about the study subjects who cut out dairy and eggs and ate a vegan diet? Did they lose enough weight to become the only dietary group in North America that's actually not overweight? Does this study conclude that populations need to cut out meat and dairy and eggs to maintain a healthy weight? The answer is, yes, only the vegans, on average, were at a healthy weight. There was a 40-pound spread between vegans and meat eaters, which is dramatic.

That said, a skeptic would be wise to probe the study's claim a little deeper—maybe the weight difference isn't explained by diet, but the fact that vegans tend to exercise more. After all, vegans by their very nature probably think about food and health more than the average American. The researchers designed their study to answer this question. They carefully measured activity levels of all groups, and, if anything, the vegans exercised less than meat eaters. But still, on average, even these slower-moving vegans were 40 pounds lighter.

What's the science behind the vegan advantage? Of course, vegetables are much less calorie dense than meat or dairy. Unless a vegan makes very bad choices, such as greasy chips and French fries, it's quite easy to eat in a healthful way. Almond milk has far fewer calories and much higher calcium levels than cow milk, for example.

One study suggests that "eating obesity" may cause obesity. Researchers of the Institute for Brain Chemistry sought to answer this question in their report, "Does Eating Obesity Cause Obesity? Dietary Predictors of Five-Year Changes in Waist Circumference."

You see, we now confine animals, genetically manipulate them, pump them up with growth hormones, and deny them exercise. Not unexpectedly, our livestock animals have become fatter—quite a bit fatter each decade. According to the USDA, a serving of chicken 100 years ago contained only 16 calories. That's half the calories of a brown rice cake. A serving of supermarket chicken today has more than 200 calories. And as the calories skyrocketed, so did the amount of fat. A serving of chicken went from less than 2 grams to 23 grams of animal fat per serving. Fifty percent more fat than a serving of ice cream. So now a chicken has 10 times more fat than a century ago, 10 times more calories, and that could explain why a chicken could be tied to our growing human belly fat. In fact, chickens themselves may be technically obese, raising concerns for animal welfare, as well as for human nutrition. Animals, of course, have become more obese, in part, to fatten up the bottom line of poultry producers. They are confined and denied exercise, while keeping food constantly available. Animals are bred based on their ability to gain weight, and then fed high-energy foods and growth hormones to promote even faster growth. All of this is a tried and true recipe for obesity.

"A chicken carcass now contains two to three times the energy coming from fat compared with protein," the study reported. "Parents may think they are still feeding their children a low-fat product, as it was in their youth, but are unknowingly feeding their children on a high-fat product."

I'll cite a few more studies that reveal why vegans are more likely to keep their weight low. The explanation begins with an interesting fact about the human body. Only one in 10 cells is human. The other 90% are bacteria. We have about 100 trillion bacterium on us or in us. The human colon, in particular, is considered the most bio-dense ecosystem in the world. It exists as a big, super-organism in a mutually beneficial, symbiotic relationship. Collectively, our gut bacteria weigh as much as one of our kidneys and is as metabolically active as our liver.

In the study, "The Microbiome and Obesity: Is Obesity Linked to Our Gut Flora?" researchers at the Scripps Clinic in La Jolla, California, examined the bacteria from feces of vegans versus meat eaters. Their rationale is that some species of bacteria are better at extracting calories from our feces than others. Pooped calories end up in the toilet rather than on our hips. Our bodies are trying to get rid of all the fecal matter, but there are certain obesity-associated bacteria in our colon that get in the way. These bacteria take our waste and break it down further and release those calories back into our bloodstream. So here our body is trying to get rid of it all, and the calories are bouncing right back.

Most of what we know about gut flora and obesity had been derived from studies on mice. We didn't really know what to think about humans. But with a 2010 Spanish study ("Gut Microbiotoa Composition Is Associated with Body Weight, Weight Gain and Biochemical Parameters in Pregnant Women"), we were given significant insight: the type of bacteria in our gut is related to body weight and weight gain. That got some researchers at the University of Vienna thinking. Maybe one of the reasons vegetarians are so much slimmer, on average, is because their diets foster more of the lean type of bacteria rather than the obese type. And that's exactly what they found. They took a bunch of fecal samples from vegetarians, did some DNA fingerprinting, compared it to omnivore feces and found significantly more of the lean type of bacteria, suggesting a smaller capacity for energy gain from food in vegetarians.

How much smaller? Perhaps 2% of the calorie intake. It doesn't sound like a lot, but it happens automatically, while we sleep even, and it adds up over time. In a year, it may come out as five pounds of fat. That may not sound like a lot either, but that's exactly how much people tend to put on annually during their mid-life years. So that could explain why vegetarians don't get that age-related weight gain that afflicts the rest of the population.

Weight loss helps explain the extraordinary explosion of resources and interest in going vegan. Never before have I seen so many major articles, in major journals, by major scientists, pleading with the world to eat less meat, whether to lose weight or stop bird flu or slow down global warming. We live in exciting times. In fact, this year, the most comprehensive attack on factory farming from a public health/infectious disease standpoint ever, the most comprehensive ever in the human scholarly record, was published.

If that's not convincing, take a look at USDA data. The number of land animals killed for U.S. consumption peaked in 2007 at 10 billion and it's been going down every year ever since. Now it's less than 9 billion, and the trend continues. Although losing meat and dairy and eggs means great things for your own body, it also does an enormous favor to the millions of animals that suffer in a confined existence with nothing to do, but stand, sleep … and eat.

The next step is to turn the page and find out how to transition into a meatless diet for a more healthful life—a life that offers up a natural feeling of energy and vitality. A life of living without the guilt of knowing your diet supports the confinement and slaughter of billions of animals. A life with a higher level of awareness and joy.

Becoming a vegan takes a little patience and planning and an enlightened mindset. But it's also a joyful way to eat, because it's the right thing to do for yourself and for the planet.

Michael Greger, MD
Creator of www.nutritionfacts. org

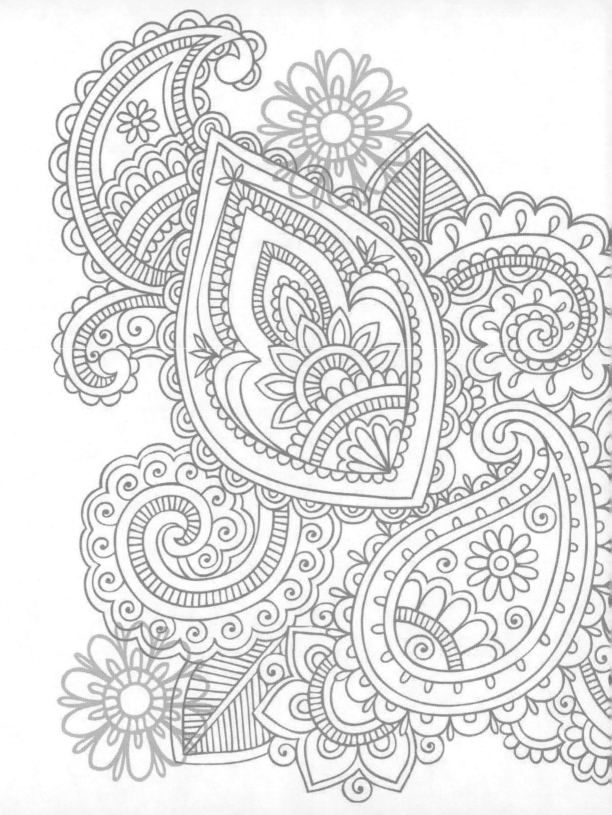

Foreword
by Dr. Mary

I love my patients. I spend four out of every seven days each week managing their health concerns, refilling their medications, and examining them. I use laboratory tests, my ears and my own two hands, searching for clues to their underlying disease. They share their most heartfelt gratitude and their deepest sorrows. They rejoice and they worry. They bring their grandchildren and dogs with them to their appointments. They know that I have time for them if they call me with a crisis on my day off, whether I'm wandering the farm market or watching my 11-year-old Ice Daughter figure skate at the rink.

After I was diagnosed with pre-diabetes five years ago, I was able to quickly turn it around with a plant-based diet. I wanted to share the incredible good health and vitality I was experiencing with my patients—the 2,000 people who rely on me to keep them healthy. I ran some ideas past a gal pal who is also a whiz-bang marketer. "That would be career suicide," she stated without a moment's consideration. Ending my career as an internist in a flaming wreck wasn't in my plans. So I kept my diet to myself for several more weeks. Problem is, you can't keep news this good to yourself.

With my newfound conviction that diet is your body's best medicine (and no side effects!), I began asking patients if they had any restrictions to their diet. But I realized that although I was well-trained to gather a patient's comprehensive surgical and family history, I had no training at all in learning about what people eat. I felt on shaky ground about how to approach the whole topic and create dietary change, so I headed to the library. (I'm guessing my co-author daughter would pick up her iPhone, but I'm a bit old school.) I discovered that food logs are notoriously unreliable. The skinniest and heaviest people keep the most inaccurate food logs, and often have no idea what they eat. The best way to determine a patient's intake is through a 24-hour food recall. Virtually everyone can remember almost exactly what they ate in the last 24 hours. This is certainly true of me. I may not remember last Monday's dinner, but the last 24 hours is still crystal clear. So I started asking everyone what they ate for breakfast, lunch, dinner, and snacks, along with what they drank.

I have limited time to work with each patient in my busy office practice. I have moments, really, with each of my patients, to determine their problem and find a suitable solution. A 24-hour food recall is the perfect tool for rapidly determining what Kris Carr refers to as the patient's Shit Pickle. Whatever is limiting them from reaching their health goals nutritionally, you'll probably find it with this tool. And while some people are unreliable in their recollection, the vast majority of people with 20 to 60 pounds to lose are repeating a few simple errors. Once corrected, they begin losing weight and feeling great. For some, the change in diet comes in small steps. As they see success and acclimate to the idea of a plant-based diet, they make more changes. Others eagerly accept the plant-based message and instantly commit to a vegan or vegetarian diet; they usually lose weight very quickly, along with all the disease baggage they've carried with it.

Now my practice is incredibly satisfying. I am able to discontinue medications virtually every day as my patients adopt healthy diets and lifestyles. I'm treating sports injuries in patients who, at one time, barely had the energy to drive back and forth to work. I've gone from seeing several patients four times a year, necessitated by their multiple chronic medical conditions, to just once a year for their annual, healthy patient screening. I'm inspired every day at the ability of these ordinary, everyday people to take my advice to heart and head in a new direction.

As I've taken this plant-based journey, I've met some great thinkers on this topic—experts who range from cutting-edge health researchers to a biologist who has spent his lifetime advocating for animal rights. They have made significant contributions to this book, and I am so grateful.

While I've enjoyed writing about health for the last two years, there are some topics that needed more time and attention than a short blog post can provide. That's why I wrote this book. I wanted to share with you all of the benefits of a healthy, cheap, easy-to-prepare plant-based diet, so you can live it up just like my fabulous patients, without the expensive office calls. I'm sharing all of my fave tricks and recipes for you to enjoy. You'll be at the doctor's office less and on the hiking trails more. You'll be seeking out a few, great local farmers who can tell you how they grew their food. And you'll have clear, radiant skin and sparkling eyes. You'll have to buy a belt to cinch up those clown pants you're wearing until you can get out to do some real shopping for sexy new clothes to complement your new, hot little figure. I'll send healthy, healing energy vibrations your way. Live it up!

I'll also share some stories about my medical practice, my personal life, and my two kids, one of whom is the co-author. Number One, as she's referred to on my blog, is literally my first-born child. We lived together in a tiny apartment for the first 12 years of her life while I completed high school, college, medical school and, finally, residency. Chelsea watched me develop my own career as an internist, and now she is developing her own as an OB/GYN in a tiny apartment of her own with her handsome husband in New York City.

Make a note here of what you ate in the last 24 hours:

_____

_____

_____

_____

_____

_____

_____

_____

_____

_____

_____

_____

Foreword
by Dr. Chelsea M. Clinton

When my mom decided to change her diet, I tried to ignore her. I may have eaten a little bit more meat and cheese just to annoy her. I didn't see why she had to be so picky about everything, and I didn't understand what the harm was in having a "balanced diet." Even though I was always attracted to healthy whole foods, I used to think that I could eat them along with unhealthy food, and they would cancel each other out. Unfortunately, my perception of what was unhealthy was lacking too. I thought anything sweet or fried was off limits, but at that time didn't consider American staples such as meat and milk to be anything but nourishing. This led to me think that I was eating unhealthy foods "in moderation", when I was actually eating a wildly unhealthy diet that was severely lacking in disease-fighting nutrients.

I see people making this mistake all of the time. It is simple to correct, as information is abundant on how fruits, vegetables and whole grains should not just exist as a side on your plate, but should overflow your entire plate at every meal, every day.

Once I got curious about my mom's diet (which was just around the time she started asking to borrow my jeans), I found it incredible how much knowledge and research existed on the benefits of eating more fruits, vegetables and whole grains. I was in my senior year of undergrad when I decided to research plant-based diets and subsequently made modifications to my diet. I felt like I always knew it was the right way to eat, and I believe most people know this deep down. The more I learned, the fewer animal products I ate. By the time I was heading to medical school, I couldn't wait to be surrounded by people that I thought would have discovered the same incredible information, or at the very least be open to receiving it and applying that knowledge to patient care. I was really bummed when nobody believed me or even seemed to care. In my four years of medical school, we had a two-hour lecture on nutrition that did at least tout the benefits of plant-based eating.

I remember looking around at everyone, expecting to see them looking at me and thinking, "She was right!" But my classmates just looked bored. I decided at that point to start a nutrition elective, and I was excited to see about forty of my colleagues showing up every week to learn about plant-based nutrition, nutrition in pregnancy, the physiologic implications of obesity, and hear testimonial from a cancer survivor who had fought his battle with the Gerson Therapy (essentially an organic vegetarian diet heavy on raw juices). The students who didn't take this elective, and potentially many other students across the country, are becoming doctors who espouse the same views of nutrition they had when they were children, when celebrities with white mustaches told them to drink milk, and their fathers told them to eat more meat to be strong. There is just no scientific evidence to support this misinformation. It is up to you to be your own advocate and seek out the most accurate information about what you can do at breakfast, lunch and dinner to redirect your health and change your life.

Now, I eat plant-based, whole foods because it's totally fun and feels good. You can make great food a part of your life effortlessly. This book is full of inspiration and evidence-based recommendations as well as tips and ideas that will have you on the right track, practically overnight. All of that great fuel will literally become part of your healthy body and you'll feel fantastic.

You can also put your mind at ease knowing that you are no longer compromising your health and longevity and condoning horrific factory farm practices with your daily meal choices. I've always loved to eat and I still do. Now I also love the way my diet makes me feel. I'm hoping the same for you!

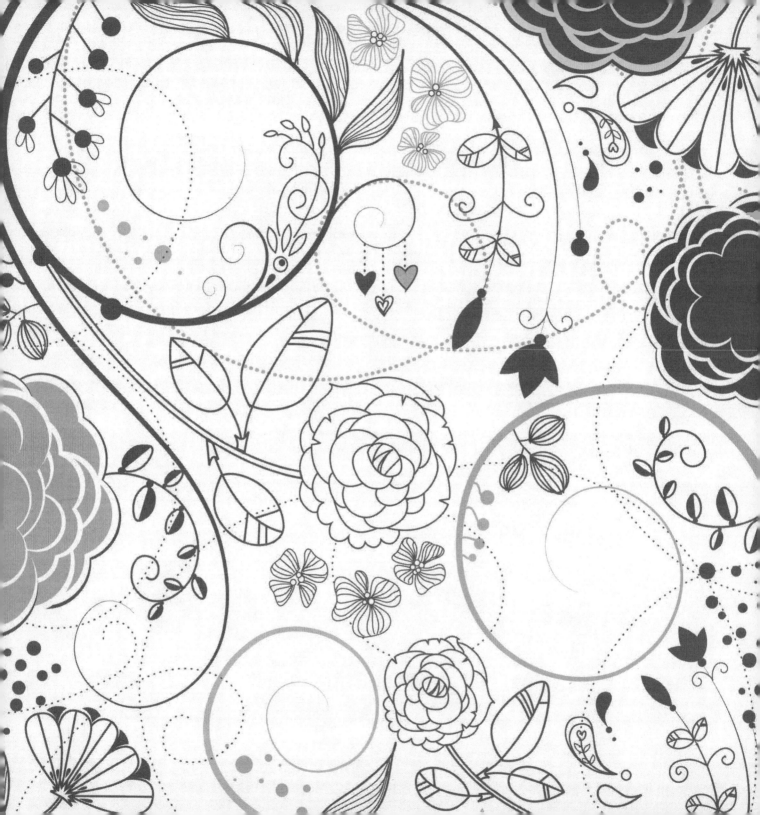

Your Pleasure, Your Addiction

— Dr. Mary —

Food always mattered to me. The lunch ladies at my parochial elementary school used to laugh when I'd ask for an extra serving of noodles, a bigger cut of the dessert cake or a little more buttered corn. Our school principal Sister Thea stationed herself at the garbage, shaking each of our individual milk containers as we returned our lunch trays. If milk remained, we were sent back to our tables to finish it. It was never a problem for me, however. I never left a drop of milk or a morsel of food behind. I ate like a dog, finished before everyone else and tore off, running out the door to claim a great location on the monkey bars for the rest of recess.

I was always going to be a scientist, once my childhood dream of becoming a nun was utterly squashed at puberty by a thousand-pound weight of hormones. I dreamed of being a bench researcher at the National Institute of Health in Maryland, studying viruses, perhaps even curing cancer. I idolized Sam Ho, *Time Magazine's* Man of the Year in 1984, awed at the depth of his knowledge of T-cells in the midst of the emerging HIV/AIDS epidemic. I was going to change the world just like Dr. Ho, or at least leave a mark.

Practicality set in after I got pregnant in my junior year of high school. I needed a job that earned a steady paycheck, and my ever-practical mother couldn't see a life of bench research leading to, well, anything. "Become a doctor," she suggested matter-of-factly. I completed my undergraduate training and was accepted to medical school. Four years later, I thought, I would be a doctor.

It didn't quite work out that way. I was halfway through my first year of medical school when I overhead fellow students discussing internships and residencies. Hmm? What were they talking about, and they *took how long?* And they were *required* to become a doctor? I don't know if I was more stunned or embarrassed that I was *just* finding out. I called my mom in a panic, but she was nonchalant. "Four or ten? What's the difference?"

The Shocking News

Fifteen years later, I found myself eight years into a private solo practice in Northern Michigan, having the time of my life. I was doing hot yoga and running five to eight hours per week, raising my kids, dating a great guy, living in paradise. I ate cereal with milk for breakfast, salad with cheese and chicken for lunch, and meat with two veggies for dinner. I went to see my doctor for my annual exam, thinking of myself as a vision of perfect health. "How are you doing it?" he asked sincerely. I listed my exercise and diet choices with pride. Ideal body weight. Perfect blood pressure.

Three days later I was in the hospital hallway outside the doctor's lounge when my doctor told me that nothing was wrong, really. Except my tests came back with elevated blood sugar and high cholesterol, and further testing was necessary to determine if I had diabetes. I told him they must have mixed up the blood samples in the lab. He laughed at me, and promised to send a lab slip.

Back at the office, I pricked my finger a thousand times over the next week. My blood sugar was always elevated, at every test. If I fasted for 12 hours and did 90 minutes of hot yoga, it would drop by about 10 points. Levels were bad before I left work in the afternoon. They weren't much worse after two cookies, which oddly made me a little angrier. They never went below 115. They often went as high as 127. Then I got really angry! Wasn't I the picture of health? And now my blood sugar revealed an underlying metabolic derangement that threatened to undo everything. A girl who's a diabetic in her 30s is facing much more serious health conditions, earlier and more intensely, than a gal with a normal metabolism. The incongruity of my self-perception and my lab results was just not logical or reasonable. I imagined myself a few decades down the road with failing vision and vascular disease, heart attacks and amputations. I tried to imagine my life with an early disability. Call me a drama queen or just a doctor with enough experience to know what diseases I wanted to avoid, but this diagnosis sent me to bed. I spent hours staring at the wall and out the window, wondering what I would look like when I was 50. I imagined saying good-bye to my sweet family a little earlier than I intended.

The bed got a little boring, and I decided I wanted a solid assessment before my emotions went farther south. So I called the endocrinologist for an expert opinion. Thankfully, after a further battery of tests, he joyfully announced that I wasn't diabetic, just prediabetic, with a 16-times increased risk of developing diabetes over the following year. I asked him what I could do for my health. "Diet and exercise," he stated. The appointment was over.

I couldn't exercise more without cutting back my hours at work, and my diet was already quite perfect, or so I thought. So I began to research my condition. Plenty of drug companies had proven that pre-diabetes could be resolved with the early use of medications. I considered pharmaceutical options for myself, but not for long. Being a doctor meant also being aware of the side effects of these various, powerful medications. There had to be a more natural alternative.

My exercise included daily walks and three to four intense runs or yoga sessions a week. Most websites and professionals confirmed my opinion that my exercise was sufficient. I tentatively looked into nutrition, but with plenty of skepticism and very little belief that making a diet change would accomplish anything at all. There were some doctors out there—at the time I wouldn't have considered them "real doctors"—suggesting a vegetarian or vegan diet for curing all kinds of diseases. Crazy. Ridiculous. No way was I going to go off the deep end and start compromising my health with a vegan diet. Where would I get my protein? What about the calcium for my skeleton?

I continued to contemplate alternatives and move through my days in a bit of a stupor. Before my diagnosis, I used to meditate while I was running, focusing on the image that I was running away from the chronic disease and illness which plagued the rest of my family. *Good health*, breathe in. *Sickness*, breathe out. I imagined myself outpacing the grim reaper. Now I was the sick one. And meditating on *that* was not empowering. Not at all.

Then I had a veg day. I wanted an egg sandwich, but I had fruit for breakfast. I had pasta for lunch, and I decided to eat veg pasta for dinner on a crazy whim, instead of a sirloin. I figured my sugar would be through the roof the next day. Instead, it was under 100 for the first time since my diagnosis. Wow. Holy cow. This couldn't possibly be happening.

So began my travels into the vegetarian landscape. I didn't come along like a gal headed for a beach vacation with my bag packed with all my favorite sundresses and two bathing suits with matching cover-ups. I came along stomping my feet and pouting, standing in front of my fridge in the middle of the night staring at the cheese, dreaming of barbecued ribs, spitting out soy milk and, overall, acting like a big fat baby who'd misplaced her pacifier.

Six months later, at my next appointment with my primary doctor, my prediabetes had resolved. My total cholesterol, which had been modestly elevated, dropped by 70 points. I told him you can get crazy, wildly healthy following this vegan diet I'm on. I told him I cured my prediabetes and cut my cholesterol 30 percent with my diet. He shook his head and laughed, then excused himself and left. I got dressed and went home, wondering what to do next.

Mastering Pleasure

At the age of 15, I was having fun and lots of other things I shouldn't have been having with my boyfriend, who was a senior in high school. We were riding dirt bikes, shooting guns, swimming and sailing in summer, and cross country skiing to each other's houses on snow days in the winter. We liked sailing on days when the weather experts warned of small craft advisories on Lake Michigan—days when the waves would crash over the hull of the sailboat, drenching us and leaving us gasping for air and checking to see if our cigarettes were still dry enough to smoke. We were rotten-little-no-good teenagers, except for our Honor Society and Sierra Club memberships, and our activity in the Thespian Society. Our mortality was miles away.

My boyfriend's mother prepared the most delicious meals, like perfect barbeque with creamy salads and tangy lemonade. I spent considerable time in the kitchen with her, because watching her cook gave me that reassuring feeling of being with an expert, someone with total understanding of the subject matter. Time melted away while she worked. The irrelevancy of time is a rare treat in our clock-obsessed world, but still observed by the master craftsmen who thrive on a good job rather than a timely one. I got the same feeling years later as I watched my favorite chemistry professor work in his lab. I still get it with a few of my colleagues as they work with a patient, sending a little shiver through me. Clearly my boyfriend's mom was a master in the kitchen, and I was in the presence of someone who knew exactly what she was doing.

Her husband came home at the usual hour, often a little grumpy, settling his lanky runner's frame into a chair by the fireplace, which may or may not have been radiating a comforting warmth, depending on the season. He'd ask for a drink, a gin and soda, and my boyfriend's mom would eventually work her way around to preparing it for him. We never drank spirits in my childhood home and this drink before dinner seemed upscale and a little forbidden. The liquor bottles at my house were relegated to an upper shelf near the cleaning supplies, taken down only when my Uncle Bill visited twice a year from Florida.

The doctor's wife got out the ice and filled the glass, then cut through a fresh lime to squeeze its contents over the ice. She then turned to face me almost full on, revealing an almost imperceptible smirk. She knew she had my full attention. She returned to the drink. With her back to the doctor and the drink well hidden from his view, she added a long, slow pour of gin to his glass. Except she held her thumb over the end of the bottle, preventing any gin from being poured. If a drop of gin dripped off her thumb after the bottle was righted, I didn't see it. She quickly filled the glass with soda and delivered it to her weary husband.

He took a long, slow drink from the glass, and immediately began to complain. "You've mixed this too strong. You've got to be more careful next time. This is way too strong. I'm only going to have one drink tonight."

Later, she explained her behavior in detail. When they were first married, her husband was a smoker. She wouldn't tolerate a smoker and immediately insisted he stop. Then he started to eat too much to compensate for not smoking, developing an unsightly bulging tummy. So she told him he ought to go for a run or something. He started running around the block a bit instead of eating away his anxieties. Now she is married to a nonsmoking, very lean, marathon runner. Controlling his consumption of alcohol, she said, was just another way of expressing her love for a man who enjoys experiencing pleasurable things.

Pleasure Is Good

In varying levels of distress, so many of my patients have asked, begged or frankly pleaded for a diet pill that will cut their appetite and make eating less pleasurable. The drug companies have been working on this magic pill for years, but every time they limit the pleasure of eating to curb appetite, they increase the risk of depression and suicide to unacceptable levels. Feeling pleasure is an important part of the experience of eating and also an important part of the experience of living. Curbing pleasurable responses to favorable stimuli and dissociating yourself from pleasure is an undesirable outcome.

Eating is an *especially* pleasurable thing. It feels good to eat, whether you are happy or sad. We should celebrate important events with shared meals, offering some of our bounty to our friends and loved ones. There is a tribal component to the shared meal, community being created by dining together, and that needs to be respected

SHOOT ME UP DUDE ... WITH SUGAR, FAT AND SALT

Sugary foods stimulate the release of the body's own opioids (morphine-like chemicals) in the brain.

Sugar and high-fat foods stimulate the brain's pleasure and reward centers through the dopamine receptors, exactly like addictive drugs.

Pharmaceutical drugs that block the brain's heroin receptors work in the same way to reduce the consumption and preference for sweetened and high-fat foods in both normal weight and obese binge eaters

and celebrated. It is not reasonable, and certainly not healthy, to separate pleasure from eating.

That's the trouble with pleasure. Certain foods have powerful addictive capacities that can overwhelm people. Studies show that chocolate milkshakes light up the same areas of the brain as cocaine, alcohol and gambling. The food industry has studied food desirability and created foods with hypernatural levels of appeal, leading to over stimulation of the pleasure centers. You, dear reader, have a food you crave, a food so delicious that you just can't resist it. Almost all of us have an irresistible treat. I'm going to guess it's not a carrot stick. It's one of these engineered industrial foods with a level of sweetness or saltiness or creaminess (or all three) that is not found in a natural whole food. A candy bar or sweet treat. A creamy latte or a buttery bakery item. A savory barbequed meat or gravy-soaked mashed potato.

When a woman routinely eats a concentrated source of fat, salt or sugar, it limits her ability to get suitable pleasure out of healthy foods. When you are regularly eating cheesecake or drinking pop, you don't really get to enjoy the sweetness in an apple or a carrot. If you're always eating chicken and red meat, you are overlooking the creaminess in beans. Healthy whole foods taste bland because the pleasure centers have been dulled from overstimulation. It's like any other pleasurable activity. It's good in small doses, but gets a little out of control if some limitations aren't placed on the behavior.

I suggest to my patients that they try using distraction to avoid falling into an unhealthy snack trap. Focus on a project or get up and do a few stretches or take a little walk, instead of searching out a snack. It takes your mind off a little hunger pang and moves you more quickly toward your personal health goals. If the urge comes back again, tackle another task, meditate or do a few push-ups. Lord knows there are a million ways to get food when you are hungry, and a huge snack industry is betting on you giving into a craving. When you pay a dollar for five cents worth of flour in a little bag of pretzels from the vending machine, the snack industry laughs all the way to the bank. Meanwhile, you despair when you try to button your jeans.

The Crave

What is the strongest, most successful way to reinforce behavior? Random, unpredictable reinforcement. It explains why people return, again and again, to pull the lever on the slot machine. If the gambler knew that the slots paid out every 50 plays, there would be no interest in the game. The interest comes from the slots paying out randomly and unpredictably. The gambler doesn't know if she's going to hit it big on the fifth pull or the fiftieth pull, and the possibility of hitting it big keeps her pulling the lever, often well past any reasonable or logical point.

Highly cravable foods interact with your brain the same way as the slot machine. You've got the brownies, the ice cream or the chocolate

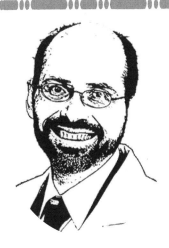

MEET COCOA, A GOOD-FOR-YOU ADDICTION ...

—MICHAEL GREGER, MD
CREATOR OF WWW.NUTRITIONFACTS.ORG

Cocoa comes from a bean, the cacao bean, and has a lot of wonderful health- promoting flavonol phytonutrients that are good for your body in a myriad of ways: they lower your blood pressure, lower bad cholesterol—and boost your good cholesterol. But wait! You've probably heard that only exercise can boost your good cholesterol. Exercise, it seems, and . . . cocoa.

Recent scientific studies of cocoa all come down to this succinct advice: "Eat cocoa." Notice I didn't write, "Eat chocolate." And milk chocolate is completely out of the question because milk blocks the positive effects in cocoa just as it does in tea.

But even dairy-free dark chocolate is made out of things you don't want—fat and sugar. The fat is saturated cocoa butter, which is one of the few plant-based fats that is actually bad for you because it raises your cholesterol. Sugar isn't good for you either. So how do you get the benefits of the cacao bean without the bad stuff? Cocoa powder. Cocoa powder has no sugar and no fat, just the incredibly-good-for-you phytonutrients.

Cocoa also unstiffens your arteries, powerfully boosts your immune system, and may even combat the effects of aging! Cacao beans and aging makes for an unexpected friendship. That is my kind of friend.

So turn your breakfast smoothie into a chocolate smoothie by adding some cocoa powder and make it even healthier. Ready for a recipe?

Chocolate Breakfast Smoothie

Dutch-process cocoa

Date sugar

Frozen dark red cherries or berries

Plant-based milk

Put all the ingredients in a blender and you have a chocolate milkshake that is actually good for you. Literally health-promoting. Meaning the more chocolate milkshake you drink, the healthier you will be. Take out the berries and heat it up for healthy hot chocolate. Or, instead of milk, add silken tofu and you have instant chocolate pudding. The more chocolate pudding you eat, the healthier you are. What can I say—nutritional science has never tasted so good!

NOTE: Date sugar is NOT sugar. It's a whole food—whole dates, just pulverized. If you can't find it locally, you can buy it online at Whole Foods.

available in the house somewhere. Perhaps you've even put it in the downstairs freezer to make it less accessible, which isn't a bad idea, but more on that later. Treating yourself with a little yummy bite of the food you particularly crave is a thought that crosses your mind many, many times each day. Maybe 100 times a day. Each time the thought crosses your mind, you play the devil/angel against each other, each of your alter egos sitting on your shoulders and whispering in your ear. The angel on your right shoulder urges you to avoid unhealthy treats. The devil on the left shoulder suggests you give into temptation, just this once. Angel wants you to stick to your plans for a healthy diet. Devil encourages you to start your healthy diet tomorrow.

All of this back-and-forth is time consuming and energy sapping. The food is avoided, or ingested, but that doesn't really matter. What really matters is that the food has been in control of your brain over the last several seconds of your life while you've fought with yourself over pleasure reinforcement. The inanimate object, usually sugar, fat, flour, meat or dairy, is leading your brain around on a leash while your poor body follows behind, leaving you with the consequences of random, unpredictable reinforcement.

For me, the addictive food is yummy coffee. I love a great cup of fair-trade, organic, shade-grown coffee with a big pour of vanilla soy

Trust Your Body
~ Anne Stanton, Health Writer and Waist Away Editor

For years, I had an uneasy relationship with food. I was skinny, yes, but didn't seem to trust myself around anything with a high calorie count. If there was ice cream in the freezer or a package of cookies in my cupboard, it didn't stay there for very long. Maybe 10 minutes after getting home. I would walk through the front door and be drawn to the cookie like a crow to road kill. I couldn't eat just one cookie. I'd eat one and then another and then another. Despite what my head told me.

This is going to sound weird, but as a business major, I had learned the law of diminishing returns and created my own theory as it applied to food. The first cookie tastes awesome. The second, third and tenth—not so much. In fact, any cookie after three simply tastes like unadulterated guilt. Even so, I would ignore both my head and stomach and gorge. One lonely night in college (freshmen year, of course), I finished off an entire package of cookies. The last one tasted like sweet sawdust. (Keebler Sandies. Haven't eaten a single one of them since then). Needless to say, I never kept desserts of any kind in the cupboard or freezer. I began to avoid baking, too.

And I loved to weigh myself. Morning, noon and night. Truthfully, my weight was on the low side—right around 122 pounds or so. But my enjoyment of food wasn't incredibly high either. Instead of pleasure, I looked at food as units of calories. I could tell you the number of calories of any food item you named. And then I could tell you how many minutes of running or racquetball or bike riding it would take to work off.

In 1991, I became pregnant with my first child, Johnny. For the first time in my life, I developed a keen desire to eat good food. I began reading cookbooks. I even started cooking complicated dishes. I finally understood what it meant to be a "foodie," even though the term wasn't around at the time. I loved this new, amped up sensation of taste, but I stressed as I gained weight—nearly 40 pounds. My doctor told me not to worry since my weight was low to begin with, but I worried anyway.

And then after I had my son, I became *really* concerned. I had an extra 20 pounds that refused to come off. Twenty pounds! I missed my trim figure. I went to buy clothes at my usual places and couldn't find a single dress that fit.

When my adorable, but colicky son, was six weeks old, I had to go back to work. My duplex neighbor, Bonnie, was unemployed at the time and needed a job. She was a quiet, loving person, so I hired her as our daycare provider. But I more than suspected she was anorexic.

Well, things clicked along for several weeks until one gray-skied week, my husband and I came down with stomach flu that carried with it a double whammy of diarrhea and throwing up. Within a week, we'd both lost five pounds. Well, we must have given the bug to baby Johnny because Bonnie called and said got the flu, too. My first thought was, poor Bonnie! She was already alarmingly skinny. She couldn't afford to lose even a pound.

A few evenings later, I drove into our shared driveway and saw Bonnie through the window. In the gloom of her kitchen light, she stood looking down at her sink. Her cheeks were sunk deep into her face. Her skin was draped over her high cheekbones to clearly reveal each and every facial bone of her skull. I was reminded of a Holocaust victim.

Continued...

And suddenly it struck me. Bonnie and so many anorexics like her had been created by our society's food obsession, the air-brushed models, the impossibly thin actresses, the Victoria's Secret catalogs. This is what anorexia looked like, I thought, and I feared Bonnie would die. She was only 42. What a tragedy to die of starvation in a country of such plenty.

I immediately called her mother, who took Bonnie to the hospital where she was hooked up to a feeding tube. I later learned that she had slipped to 82 pounds. With so little left on her 5'6 frame, she was precariously close to death.

As I gazed at Bonnie through the window that night, my obsession with food slipped away. I consider myself a spiritual person, and I realized I was *born* with the natural gifts of hunger and satiety. *Gifts* because I realized that if I trusted my own body and appetite, weight would never be an issue again. I didn't need, and never needed a scale. I threw it away.

So my mantra became *trust*. I would simply trust in what my appetite was telling me. My one rule of eating became this: eat when hungry, don't eat when full. If I wanted a cookie, I would eat one, no big deal, no big guilt trip. I'd just remind myself that sugar wasn't the kind of toxin I wanted in my body. Once I gave myself over to my natural appetite, eating became downright joyful. I began cooking again with gusto and savored every wonderful bite!

Soon, I was back down to 122 pounds. Now, 20 years later, I weigh 125 pounds. I'm seemingly unaffected by the lower metabolism that's supposed to hit in middle age (I'm 55), and I would argue that's because I eat a largely plant-based diet and I love to exercise.

So basically, my advice is this: don't second-guess your hunger pangs, even if they wake you up at 2 a.m. in the morning. Even if you feel weirdly full at dinner after just a few bites. Just go with what you *really* feel and see what happens.

creamer from my local organic food store. It sounds pretty harmless, except that it is really so delicious that I can't drink enough of it, and I find myself drinking a large coffee every afternoon. We can debate the merits of coffee all day, but this high-fat, sugary habit of mine was impacting my health and my pocketbook.

So I put the coffee on a schedule. I decided that if I bring my reusable shopping bags when I'm doing my Saturday shopping, I get to have a cup of coffee. At first, I wasn't consistent with my shopping bags, and I missed the treat a few times. Those were some very bad days. Then I started to leave the reusable bags in the car, and now I virtually never miss out on my treat. It is such a pleasure to sip that cup of coffee while I shop for all my household stuff! Since I'm not treating myself all the time, the pleasure of the treat is intensified even more when I get the opportunity to enjoy it. When you schedule

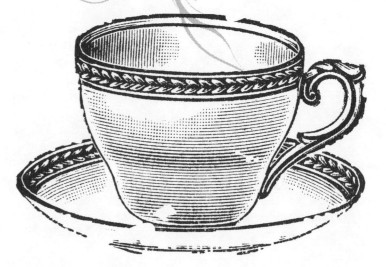

your treat, you remove the inconsistency, and the treat loses a tremendous amount of power. When you start the time-wasting process of deciding whether or not you will have the treat, you can stop it almost immediately by reminding yourself that the treat is scheduled every Saturday morning, for example. Choose whatever day and time make the most sense so you can get the most out of your treat. Then, with the treat in its proper place, you can move your mind to other things, like your relationship with your chosen partner, your children or your parents, or you can think about the great new barrette you saw on Etsy.com.

The Addiction

Sometimes a treat is more than just a treat, however. Sometimes a food has such a powerful influence that is needs to be managed a little differently. For old Dr. Mary, it was the barbecued ribs. My former boyfriend, and still a dear friend, the Tall Texan, truly makes the best ribs of anyone, ever. I know y'all think you've had some stellar ribs, but you'll just need to come on up here to Northern Michigan and visit. If you come visit me in the most beautiful place in the United States http://abcnews. go.com/Travel/best_places_USA/sleeping-bear-dunes-michigan-voted-good-morning-americas/story?id=14319616 , you will find the landscape rich with rolling hills, deep blue water and hot sandy beaches. In the winter, it's wise to bring an extra layer of warm clothing so you can enjoy the quiet, leafless forests on snowshoes or cross-country skis, then cuddle with your honey by a crackling fire with a cup of cocoa after your excursion, listening to the wind whistle you a little melody.

You'll also find the Tall Texan on his back porch overlooking Lake Michigan, coaxing the smokiest, sweetest, tangiest flavor out of his pork ribs. When they are done, 12 hours after the process is started, they are irresistible. I've eaten them until I've been quite sick, full to the brim. I've embarrassed myself in front of company, covered with sauce and grease and bent over my plate. When I made my dietary change, the ribs were the food I missed the most. I knew that even tasting a rib would take me completely off my new plant-based diet and in a bad direction that would be extremely hard to correct.

So I didn't eat a single bite of ribs for two years. After about six months, I felt the grip of this food loosening, and by two years, well, now I can take ribs or leave ribs. Breaking an addiction is a two-year process. Stopping the behavior is quick and relatively effortless. It is the rebuilding of the circuitry in the central nervous system that takes the time. If you have this relationship with a particular food, you may want to consider total cessation instead of just scheduling your treat. In some cases, it is reasonable to try to find an alternate choice for the foods you are craving. In other cases, that's about as reasonable as suggesting that a crack addict have just a tiny bit of crack every day.

Some of my patients have serious addictions to alcohol. I don't know if it is brain chemistry

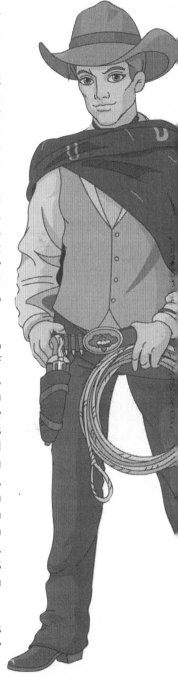

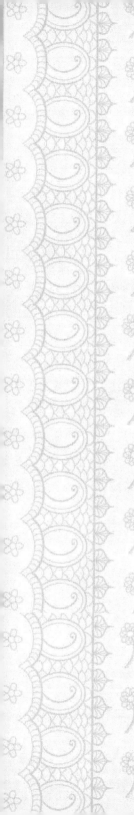

or metabolism, but one drink leads to another, and these poor patients are lost in an abyss of alcoholism. Most of my patients who misuse alcohol can curb their use and modify the ingestion to a reasonable amount, still enjoying the product without consuming excessively. They are scheduling their treat.

You need to make an honest assessment of where you are at with your problem foods. Your problem food may be able to be scheduled, like my coffee, leaving you feeling in control and on track with your overall goals. Your problem food could be like my Tall Texan ribs, so delicious that you are truly out of control when you get around it. In that case, girl, you'd better watch out. You better stay miles away from that food until you feel its grip loosen, or you may find yourself off track all over again after you take that first bite. But most of the time, it's just a matter of scheduling the treat.

Working Your Pleasure

Addiction and pleasure are next door neighbors, but seeking pleasure and experiencing pleasure doesn't have to have such a bad name. People with addictive personalities seek pleasure and often they will work very hard to achieve their desired outcome. Frequently, people who have addictive personalities are able to channel their desire for pleasure into stressful work situations. Because people with addictive personality tendencies are interested in working hard to achieve the desired

outcome, they are often quite successful in work environments, as long as they continue to channel their energies toward seeking pleasure in healthy ways.

Finding joy in exercise and great food is another way to channel those pleasure-seeking tendencies. Find your most pleasurable, healthiest activities and start to pursue them in earnest. Pretty soon, you'll be the lean marathon runner with a body that is the envy of all your friends, just like my boyfriend's mom.

And don't forget about all the lovely, pleasurable pastimes that don't involve food. Sometimes the most pleasurable things are very simple. Instead of popping into the kitchen when the next urge hits you, think of the baboons you've seen picking the nits off each other in the jungle. There's no need to do that, but grooming yourself or your partner can take the place of eating without leaving you feeling deprived. Try giving yourself a pedicure, brushing your hair or applying some moisturizing lotion to your arms and legs before heading to the kitchen. You'll be more in touch with your gorgeous bod after the grooming. The pleasant sensations that come with grooming will also release plenty of dopamine to stimulate the pleasure centers in your brain, leaving you feeling really good without the consequences of eating something really bad. Maybe the advice to brush your hair a hundred times before going to bed prevented a lot of binge eating.

Get the Board Members on Your Side

~ Anne Stanton, Health Writer and Waist Away Editor

I once interviewed my favorite therapist, Greg Holmes, about the troubling conundrum of why people *know* how important it is to exercise, but don't do it. Perhaps even more important than weight loss, exercise keeps your bones healthy. But still, so many women avoid exercise like a bad cold. Why? Dr. Holmes has a theory. Everyone has a "board of directors" in their brain. This so-called board ponders and then decides all your life's decisions. When it comes to exercise, the conversation might go like this:

Board Member 1: You NEED to exercise. It's GOOD for you! And summer will be here in a month.

Board Member 3: Aggghhhh summer! My legs look like stuffed German sausages! That does it. I'm *going* to the gym."

Board Member 2: But what about the dear, sweet children. I already don't spend enough time with them. And now I'm talking about taking an *hour* in the gym? Three times a week? That's just so selfish of me.

Board Member 1: But I can't hike with them because it makes me breathe like Darth Vader. I've got to do *something*.

Board Member 2: But not running. Gawd, not running. It's *no fun."*

It's that last one—no fun—that often stops the discussion cold. Your board of directors will rule "no" every time. So what Dr. Holmes is getting at is this: when it comes to exercise, choose what you love to do—ice skating, tennis, running, maybe skiing or bicycling. And then do it often. It won't be hard because you'll return to the memory of feeling happy, of feeling proud of your muscles feeling tingly and alive all day long.

If you haven't exercised in awhile, start easy with walking. Get some great music and lose yourself in your favorite songs. If you find yourself coming up with excuses at the last minute, make a "date" with a friend, particularly a friend who is reliable and doesn't cancel at the last minute. Walking with a friend beats going to a smoky bar. Your friendship will deepen and you'll love the long, uninterrupted conversations. Your board members will be sure to take note.

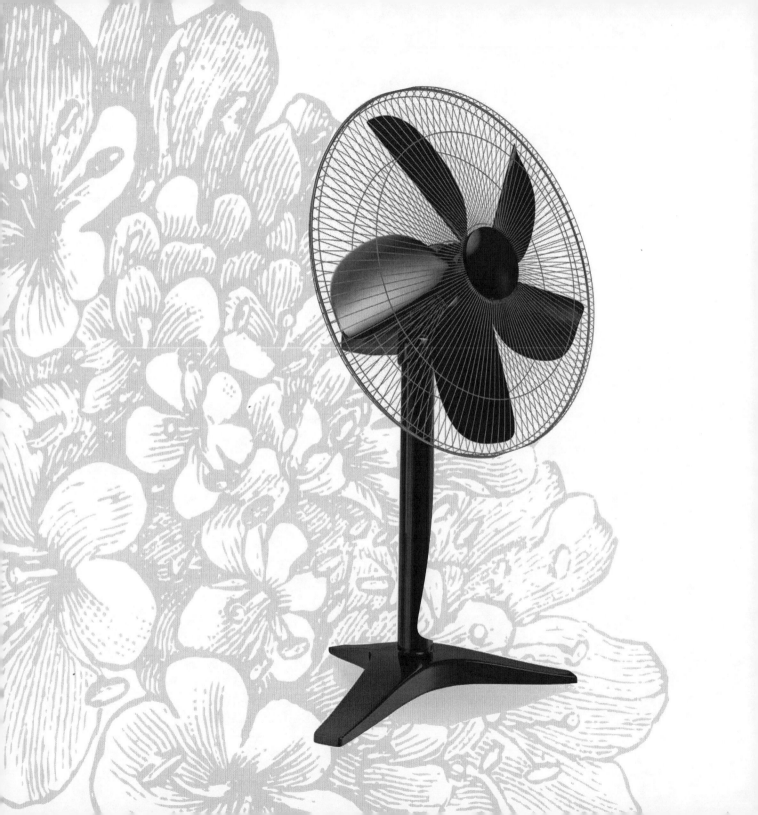

Let a Plant-Based Diet Cool You Down

— Dr. Mary —

After withdrawing from animal products abruptly and completely six years ago, I developed drenching night sweats. I woke up wet and slimy like a fish, and often switched to the guest bedroom to finish my night's sleep, since my bed was rendered uninhabitable. I thought my metabolism had gotten completely boggled, and the next step would be an early and untimely death after a hip fracture or some other horrible outcome reserved for the very sick and very old. I wondered what kind of witchcraft was leading a gal in her late 30s to be drenched in sweat in the middle of the night.

$\mathcal{B}$ut after just a few short weeks, my body balanced out beautifully. I experienced less backache and cramping with menses, clearer thinking and a higher level of energy. I chalked up the night sweats to bad dreams. It was years later before I made the connection.

Your Hot Flash

Eighty percent of women experiencing their transition to menopause are symptomatic in one way or another. These symptoms, fortunately, decrease as we get older. By the age of 55, only 6.6 percent of women will still suffer persistent hot flashes and night sweats. By the age of 65, only 3.4 percent of women are still having vasomotor instability, the

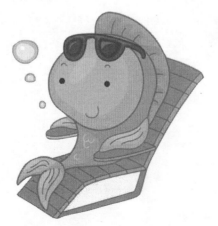

medical term for hot flashes and night sweats. These are the women who may benefit from the addition of hormone replacement therapy to control their symptoms if they are perceived as life-altering or intolerable.

Hot flashes and night sweats are increasingly well-studied, but poorly understood. Sensors applied to women's chests failed to identify actual temperature differences in women suffering from hot flashes, thus failing to prove that temperature dysregulation is the cause. The bottom line is, after years of study in multiple universities, we still don't know exactly what causes a hot flash.

But we do have some clues as to what's happening. The hypothalamus is responsible for temperature regulation, and, as you might have guessed, it has plenty of estrogen receptors on it. Interestingly, the hypothalamus also has plenty of testosterone receptors. Our ovaries make estrogen, but they also make testosterone. Lower levels of both testosterone and estrogen after menopause may contribute to temperature dysregulation. Both of these sex hormones occur naturally in women, but at declining levels as women age. A woman can expect a decline of about 50 percent in the levels of her hormones from the age of 20 until 40. From age 40 to the average menopausal age of 50, women see further reductions in estrogen. Before the actual onset of menopause, it's not uncommon for women to suffer hot flashes prior to their periods, when estrogen levels are at their lowest in their menstrual cycle.

Estrogen is naturally present in every woman's body. The term "estrogen" really refers to a group of hormones, including estrone, estradiol, and others. We will refer to this group of hormones as estrogens. Studies have identified different physiological characteristics with different estrogens, but that is a subject for a different book. Before menopause, ovaries make estrogen, but many other cells are also capable of manufacturing estrogen. In fact, you can think of fat cells as little estrogen factories, efficiently converting hormones produced in the adrenal glands into estrogens.

While women have estrogen receptors in their breast tissue, they also have estrogen receptors in many other cells of the body, including the skeleton, brain and even the kidneys and adrenal glands. The effects of estrogen on many of the organs is still not clearly defined, and I don't know if scientists will ever determine the function of some estrogen receptors. We do know that estrogen is, at different times of the life cycle and at different concentrations, both valuable to some organs and problematic for others. While estrogen is valuable in growing breast tissue in the adolescent female, it is detrimental to many women recovering from breast cancer. When researchers add a little bit of estrogen to cancer cells in the laboratory, cancer cells grow much faster. In fact, many modern pharmaceuticals used for treating breast cancer work to reduce the ability of available estrogen to stimulate cancer cells by blocking the receptor or by limiting the body's ability to synthesize estrogen at all.

Your News Flash

Diet controls estrogen levels too. National Cancer Institute data shows that when a woman begins a high-fiber, low-fat diet, estrogen levels can drop by 15 to 50 percent. A woman following a plant-based diet will still have plenty of estrogen to support necessary functions at the molecular level, but there will be far less estrogen available to stimulate tumor growth. That sounds like a good thing for cancer prevention.

A study published in 2003 by the Journal of the National Cancer Institute found that when girls, ages eight to ten, reduced the amount of fat in their diet, their estrogen levels decreased to lower and safer levels. By increasing the consumption of whole grains, beans, fruits and vegetables, these girls dropped their estrogen levels by 30 percent compared to the girls who changed nothing. Cancer scientists believe that most cancers start small and grow over many years until they develop into a problematic tumor, and many cancer scientists think that most breast cancers originate in the adolescent breast. This is the time of life when the breast tissue is dividing most rapidly. It is in the times of rapid cellular division that DNA is most likely to divide in an irregular way. Statistically, a higher number of divisions result in a higher number of errors. When these abnormal divisions are stimulated by higher levels of estrogen, it is like fertilizing the lawn. The aberrant cell is more inclined to grow and get a good foothold with estrogen stimulation. This is why it's so vitally important to your daughter's lifelong health to consume plant foods during her adolescence. You may literally be saving her life by protecting her from the initiation of a breast cancer in her adolescence that will eventually threaten her adult life.

Overdoing Your Estrogen

In certain Asian countries, there are no words in the language to describe hot flashes or night sweats. I've always thought this was because women were undervalued in some countries, and, therefore, their concerns trivialized. If people didn't listen to women value value what women said, why would there be a broad vocabulary to describe signs and symptoms of diseases that are limited to women?

It is possible, and more likely, however, that their healthy plant-based diets attenuate the estrogen withdrawal symptoms of menopause and lead to far fewer signs and symptoms, such as hot flashes and night sweats.

Journal of National Cancer Institute data shows that girls who remove animal products from their diet experience a 30 percent decline in serum estrogen levels. I think I personally experienced relative estrogen withdrawal when I awoke as a slimy wet fish six years ago. Reducing the animal content of my diet from 40 percent of my daily calories to less than 5 percent virtually overnight resulted in a relative estrogen

deficiency, and undoubtedly, my body was aware of the change. That 40 percent reduction in estrogen in my bloodstream led to vasomotor instability and left me standing, shivering and boggled, next to my cold wet bed in the middle of the night. I'm so thankful I learned the truth about animal foods and changed my diet before that excess estrogen caused a lot more trouble. Now, I have enough estrogen to live as a healthy woman, but not so much that I'm undoing my health.

This Too Will End

The majority of women experience the menopausal transition at 50 years old. By the age of 54, virtually every woman will have completed her menopausal transition. Twenty percent of women have no signs or symptoms associated with their menopause, except cessation of the menstrual period. The other 80 percent of women are symptomatic in one way or another. The conglomeration of symptoms experienced by each individual woman seems to be related to a mixture of genetics and lifestyle.

Often, in the midst of acute symptomatic estrogen withdrawal, women can experience difficulty concentrating or increased anxiety or depression. This leads many women to arrive at my office with a request for hormonal supplementation for their perceived cognitive impairments.

While I have plenty of sympathy for someone who is feeling frustrated by depression or anxiety limiting their level of function, I can also offer plenty of reassurance. Many studies have reviewed the data on mood disorder surrounding menopause, and the results are very comforting. It turns out that when you awaken a woman several times a night with sweats and give her hot flashes all day, she's not going to be at the top of her game. Scientists have studied this problem by comparing the level of function of 60-year-old women with their fourth grade report cards. Scientists wanted to determine if a woman's mental capacities and mood were impacted by estrogen withdrawal. It turns out that the level of productivity and basic personality of the 60-year-old women studied was surprisingly consistent with the behaviors documented in the fourth grade report cards. That is, the women's personalities were quite similar to the way they had been in their childhoods, regardless of the intensity of the mood disorders surrounding their menopausal transitions.

You can learn a lot about a person by reviewing their fourth grade report card, since personality traits are well-established by that time. Conversely, you don't learn anything by watching a woman suffer through a particularly symptomatic menopausal transition, except perhaps how she will respond to stress and acute illness. If there is some difficulty concentrating or a mood disorder like depression or anxiety, it will go away once the transition is completed and the woman adjusts to her new hormonal environment.

Estrogen and Your Brain

The literature is divided on the effect of estrogen on the aging brain. While the North American Menopause Society thinks that estrogen offers minimal protection of healthy brain function, there is still considerable debate on the topic. There is not enough evidence to suggest that women supplementing with estrogen in her post-menopausal years are protecting their brains. Any small effect of estrogen withdrawal seen at the time of menopause on cognitive function is largely mitigated with the passage of time and distancing oneself from the acute situation.

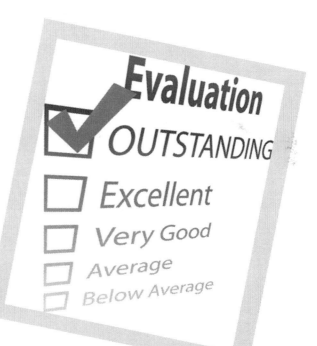

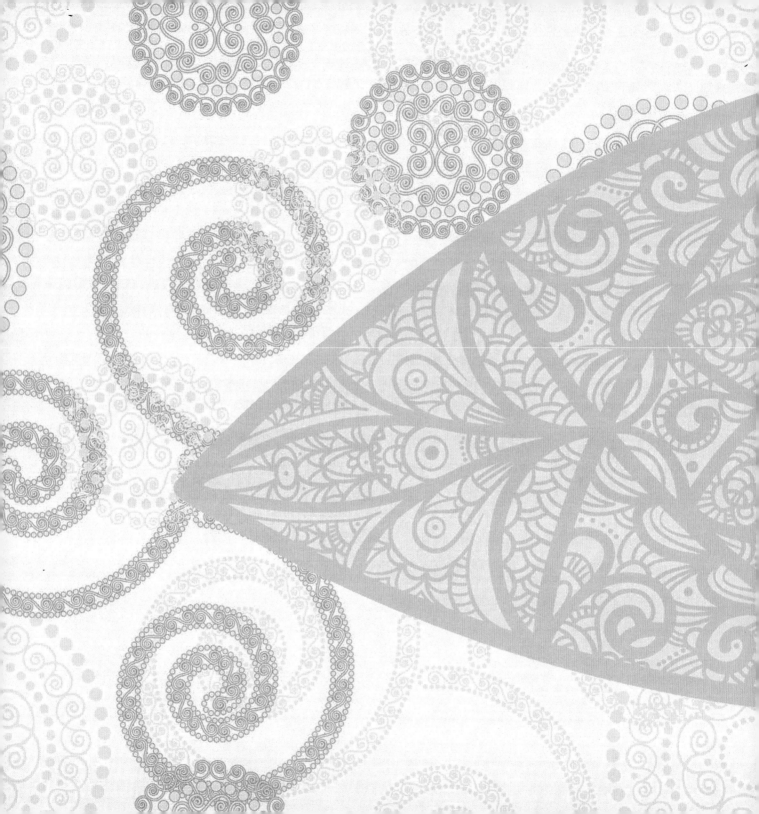

Fifty Shades of Green
Dr. Mary & Dr. Clinton

Some of my patients thoroughly enjoy their sexuality, from their teen years until well into their eighties. Yet many suffer a dramatic decrease in their desire for sex as they near menopause and fear their sex life is over. Sure it's nice not to have to worry about pregnancy and periods, but who wants to spend the rest of her life feeling like an asexual creature?

*I*f you are experiencing a flagging sex drive, you're not alone. Decreased sexual desire affects 30 percent of American women sometime in their lives, making it the most common sexual complaint. It doesn't really have to be this way, at least in most cases. There are about a million reasons why a woman should work to enhance her sexual relationship with her partner, but I'll just share the most selfish top eight with you here:

1. Physical intimacy improves mood through decreasing stress and promoting relaxation. Researchers in Scotland studied 24 women who kept records of their sexual activity. They subjected the study participants to stressful situations and monitored their physiologic responses. They found that people who had regular sexual intercourse had less blood pressure elevation in response to stress, compared to those who engaged in other sexual behaviors, or abstained from sex. Another study published in the same journal, *Biological Psychology*, found that frequent intimacy was associated with lower diastolic blood pressure in cohabitating participants.

2. People engaging in sex once or twice a week have better immunity. Scientists at Wilkes University in Pennsylvania compared saliva samples of 112 college students. Based on their reported frequency of sexual activity once or twice a week, students were found to have higher levels of immunoglobulin A, or IgA, which is important for protection against infection. This antibody is found is high concentrations in the saliva and is considered a first-line of defense against colds and other upper respiratory infections.

3. Sex burns your ass. It takes a little work to do it well. Thirty minutes of sex burns 85 calories or more. Remember that one pound is 3600 calories. Twenty-one hour-long sessions will burn a pound. It's no wonder my patients don't gain weight when they go on vacation without the kids!

4. Sex is good for your cardiovascular health. Researchers in England found that having sex twice or more per week reduced the risk of fatal heart attack by half for men, compared with those who had sex less than once a month. Results of the 20-year study of 914 men were published in the *Journal of Epidemiology and Community Health*.

5. Doing a little pelvic floor exercise during sex increases the pleasure, but it also strengthens the area and reduces problems with urinary incontinence. It's easy to do: tighten the muscles of your pelvic floor as though you are stopping the flow of urine, count to three, then release. Repeat until you've done ten, or until you've got your man going out of his mind.

6. Sex helps you sleep better. True that. Apparently the oxytocin released during orgasm promotes sleep directly, but lovers are also awash in plenty of other feel-good hormones like serotonin and dopamine. In addition, a good night's sleep offers the added benefits of healthy blood pressure and more success at maintaining your healthy weight. So don't take it personally when your guy is into you at 10 p.m. and asleep at 10:01 p.m. It's just the oxytocin.

7. Oxytocin, the hormone released with orgasm, also reduces pain, primarily through secondary release of endorphins. In the *Bulletin of Experimental Biology and Medicine*, 48 volunteers were asked to inhale oxytocin vapor. Then they were asked to rate their level of pain after a finger was pricked by a pin. Volunteers who inhaled oxytocin vapor lowered their pain thresholds by half when compared to controls. So don't be surprised if your headache or arthritis actually feel better after sexual intercourse. Researchers in North Carolina and Pittsburgh (Grewen, K. M., Girdler, S. S., Amico, J. & Light, K. C.) found that even hugging your partner resulted in increasing levels of oxytocin.

8. Finally, sex improves your self-esteem. While some people with high levels of self-esteem report that they have sex to feel even better, others report that having loving, connected sex gives flagging self-esteem a needed boost.

What the Science Says

So let's start with the question of aging and sex. Is there evidence that getting older brings with it an automatic decline in your sex life? Or is something else at work? Masters and Johnson were breakthrough scientific investigators in the area of human sexuality in the 1970s when they worked and published their studies. The studies had limitations, particularly the fact that many of the participants were involved in the sex industry. Although that naturally limits the generalization of the data across the population, the data elucidate many of the normal sexual functions surrounding arousal for both women and men. Indeed, the work of Masters and Johnson laid the foundation for decades of sexual research that expanded upon their initial findings.

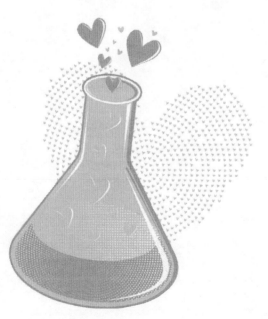

One delightful fact arising from their research was that the peak of sexuality of women occurs in their 40s. While men are thought to peak in their sexual function in their late teens, women peak much later. This puzzling statistic has left more than one medical student a little boggled in their advice to the aging female and sexuality.

Peak Sex

Let's look a little closer. For the purposes of this study, peak sexual performance was defined as the shortest time from onset of sexual stimulation to orgasm. Specifically, the shorter the time it took for the participant to achieve orgasm after stimulation, the better his or her sexual performance. By this measure, women peak at age 40, while men peak at age 18 or so. I'm not sure about you, but I think a man's peak sexuality would be better measured as the longest period of the time that he can undergo stimulation without achieving orgasm. Certainly, a man who can tolerate only a very short period of stimulation before orgasm is less desirable than a man who can wait a while and enjoy many minutes of coupling intimacy together. With that in mind, isn't it reasonable to conclude that men and women are not so poorly matched sexually as we had previously been led to believe? After all, a gal who quickly reaches orgasm coupled with a man who is able to wait awhile, sounds like a perfect combination.

Where does your diet fit into all of this? Let's turn again to Masters and Johnson and their landmark 1960 paper, *The Human Female: The Anatomy of Sexual Response,* for a little health education. In this paper, the scientists describe the successful stimulation of the human female, and the generalized physiological responses that occur. Frankly, just reading their research is a little stimulating.

In the breasts, nipple erection is the first indication of sexual excitement, with subsequent swelling of the entire areola that can partially obscure the erect nipple. The breasts increase in size by a fifth to a quarter over their normal baseline size. In the external pelvis, enlargement of the clitoris by two or three times if frequently observed. The labia majora also double or triple in size, in addition to flattening laterally to make the vaginal outlet more available to the mounting process. (I love how these researchers refer to sexual intercourse as the mounting process, presumably in the same pattern of existing research on animal sexuality.) At peak sexual stimulation, there is also a marked change in appearance to the labia minora, which turn almost burgundy red as the impending orgasmic experience approaches.

Internally, the vagina begins the process of lubrication. Coming from the walls of the vaginal barrel itself, it begins almost immediately after the onset of sexual stimulation. A telltale sign of sexual excitement is the appearance of a measle-like rash over the chest and upper abdomen. This sexual flush is more obvious in blonde or redheaded females than brunettes.

Healthy sexual responsiveness in women—and in men, for that matter—requires a healthy vascular tree, or, to put it in simpler terms, a healthy blood flow. That's because the normal responses to sexual stimulation involve engorging organs and tissues in the body with blood by the process of vasocongestion. As you and your partner get warmed up, arteries that deliver blood to the sexual organs dilate, allowing them to deliver even larger amounts of blood to the desired area. Meanwhile, veins that ordinarily drain the blood away from the tissues also dilate so that blood pools in the affected area, which effectively slows blood flow away from the tissues. This pooling creates the swelling and congestion that is seen in a normal sexual response.

As an example, if you narrow the diameter of a pipe just a little bit, you dramatically decrease the amount of fluid you are able to move through that pipe. Imagine the big straw you get in your drink at a restaurant, and how much fluid you are able to drink through that large tube. Now, imagine drinking your beverage through your coffee stirrer, the little red straw with the teeny tiny holes. You can't drink much liquid at all!

The same goes for the blood vessels feeding your sexual organs, and your male partner's sexual organs too. The extra fat you eat lines your abdominal cavity, but it also, unfortunately, lines the blood vessels that feed your heart and your brain. In addition, it lines the blood vessels that feed your breasts, vagina and your partner's sexual parts. Decreasing the diameter of the straw just a little bit decreases the flow through the tube dramatically, limiting the ability of the tissues to vagocongest and limiting a hearty sexual response.

Eating a healthy, low-fat, plant-based diet strips the arteries and blood vessels of any fatty accumulation and leaves the pipes wide open. We also know that this healthy diet will reduce your risk for chronic diseases and obesity, reduce depression and pain from arthritis. All the way around, a great plant-based diet makes a person a much better bed partner.

Now that we're on the subject of a bountiful blood flow, I'll mention that e-word, and I'm not talking erotic. I'm talking exercise. When you move your body vigorously for at least 30 minutes, you get your blood flowing and your nervous system firing. So when you schedule a vigorous walk, a game of tennis or a bike ride with your partner, leave some time afterward to rev up your body even more!

Doing the Job

Let's put health, hormones, and dilating blood vessels aside for a minute and talk about the common culprit of a fading sex life. That would be life: the buzz-killers of stress, lack of time, self-image, kids, and maybe even your own personal viewpoint on sexuality and aging.

Many married couples find their relationship lagging after years of managing the household, work, children, budget and their own personal lives. Less and less attention and energy are focused on the relationship as expectations at work intensify and partners become more preoccupied with activities and projects outside the home. Children provide a great source of satisfaction and pride for a couple, but they're also a remarkable distraction. With extended family and friends, holidays and school events, the diversions for a couple's attentions are endless, and the time and attention available to focus on the relationship shrink dramatically. It's easy to take each other for granted and even and grow resentful of each other. It's also easy to forget how valuable your partner can be when you yourself feel completely swamped and overwhelmed. That may sound a little obvious, but it's true and it's a big killer of intimacy. You remember what it was like when you were in a new relationship with your fella? All of the attention and interest was very satisfying and reinforcing. Distraction can be very detrimental to romance.

Complicating adult sexuality is the evaporation of available time opportunities, often due to the presence of teens in the home. Young children go to bed at predictable hours and wake up in the morning at a reliable time. As our offspring move into their teen years, their circadian rhythms shift, resulting in a pattern of staying up late into the night and sleeping in until the late morning. This new pattern is established as a teenager and often doesn't fully return to a more normal pattern until the child reaches his or her mid-twenties. Unfortunately, that means limited opportunity for sexuality for you and your hubby. The old opportunity to tuck the kids into the bed and hit the sack for an hour of lovemaking before falling deeply asleep with your spouse evaporates. To complicate matters further, those adolescent children also have a budding awareness of human sexuality and super sharp hearing skills, further limiting opportunities for great sex for the team that is providing the roof over their head.

Once the kids get their driver's licenses and their own transportation, their coming and goings become even more erratic. It is hard not to feel a little resentful of increasingly independent teenagers when they shrink the time and environment available for a noisy, rambunctious night with hubby, leaving sexual opportunities for vacation and days off from work. Rescheduling time for sexuality makes it easier to get around inquisitive children and other such barriers, but it's tricky when the increasing work demands of midlife put the squeeze on a couple's energies during the day. Squeezing in a nooner sounds fun, but, in reality, getting the couple back home in the midday, given commutes and noontime errands, is probably even harder than getting the couple to turn off their computer and televisions and focus on each other at night. Limited time makes for limited opportunities. On top of that, you also need a good night's sleep to maximize productivity and fend off daytime fatigue. My advice is to find a place in your schedule when you can fit in a romantic interlude— Saturday and Sunday mornings, for example, when the family is sleeping in. Treat it like a doctor's appointment. No excuses!

What Are You Doing in There?

Finally, some women have a negative perception of sexuality and aging. When we were kids, it was seriously gross when Mom and Dad would lock the door to their bedroom and get up late on Sunday. Honestly, what could they possibly be doing in there, that they needed to lock the door? Eeeeew. I'm still convinced that my own parents only had sex for procreation. Now, I'm the creepy grownup who is still interested in having sex with my partner.

If you have a notion in your mind that sexual encounters are reserved for young people, and your partner feels differently, it may be time to think about that for a while. It's reasonable to have any opinion you would like about adult sexuality. The problem arises when your partner has a different opinion, and two of you are clashing a bit under the covers. It might be worth exploring your mind for this negative connotation to adult sexuality and deciding if that idea is worth modifying.

Your Beautiful Bod

One problem might be how you perceive your body. Feeling sexual with a less than perfectly desirable body is the real trick to healthy sexuality. Estrogen levels decrease in your forties and fifties, causing extra weight to redistribute to the upper arms and abdomen, and away from the gluteal-femoral region. The result? Flat-butt, sticky-outy tummy and jigglers on the arms. Yikes. Even if there isn't extra weight redistributing, the thinning of the collagen layer of the skin, with resultant fine lines and wrinkles, can challenge even the most self-assured aging adult. We strive for the youthful perfection of the ultra-thin models glorified in our magazines, even though they are really just ultra-airbrushed imaginary images of people.

So, yes, it's hard to believe that your partner is not desirous of an airbrushed fantasy girl rather than that ordinary human being he is sleeping with each night. In reality, however, your man is in bed with you because he chooses to be. In many cases, men care more about the frequency of sexual encounters than any other key factor. That's not breaking news: men want women to put out more. And your man wants you to do whatever you need to do that makes you feel sexy and desirable. There are a number of things that heighten desirability besides honing a perfect body. Identify something you like to do that makes you feel sexy. Maybe it's dancing. Maybe you like to wear something pretty to bed. Maybe it's getting a great blowout for your hair now and then. Maybe you like to create something, like renovating a room or writing or changing your career.

Make sure you do something regularly that makes you feel sexy and attractive, and your availability for sex with your partner will certainly increase. That includes following your new, healthy, plant-based diet, which is associated with decreased rates of obesity.

Just adding some attention and interest back into a relationship can reignite passion. If you'd like to spark some flames with your partner, remember what used to excite you when you first met. If you used to enjoy going to the movies, hiking, or four-wheeling, add that fun activity back into your relationship with your partner. If you used to go sailing, see if you can find money in the budget to buy or rent a sailboat. If not, maybe your great guy would like to go for a walk on the beach. A new or familiar ritual, when practiced regularly, quickly becomes routine. Cultivate a culture within your relationship of listening with attention, and not judgment, to your partner. Remember why you fell in love with him. Going back to old favorites often helps things move forward in an exciting new, but still familiar, direction.

STEAMY READS EQUAL STEAMY WINDOWS

If you find that you're arriving to the party feeling flat, then it's time for a little inspiration. Pull out your hubby's treasure trove of *Playboys* or soft porn flicks. You might only need a few minutes of watching, say, two women seducing each other before you turn it off and start your own action.

We also recommend stocking up on the new "Mommy porn" novels. There's a reason *Fifty Shades of Grey* is a huge hit. It offers up sex scenes almost as fast as you can turn the pages. There's a whole lot we don't like about the book—the pedestrian writing and the unrealistic expectations for sex. A virgin who has three earth-shaking orgasms the first time out? But the worst aspect is the question driving the plot: can an innocent, virgin girl heal a damaged-goods, rich and handsome guy who gets off on hurting and disciplining her. Still, it offers a bazillion ideas for new sex adventures (blindfolds, nipple orgasms, the thrill of never knowing what's around the corner). Billionaire Christopher Grey might have his issues, but he does put a lot of thought into turning on girlfriend Anastasia Steele.

Fifty Shades will get you hot, but it feels like fast food erotica—no depth with a bit of a guilty aftertaste. There are lots of other romantic reads that will leave both your brain and body feeling

hot and satisfied. Some erotic oldies, but goodies include Gael Greene's 1970's classic erotic novels *Blue Skies, No Candy* and *Doctor Love*. Anaïs Nin delivers great sex scenes along with unexpected plot twists. And who can forget Erica Jong's *Fear of Flying* and D.H. Lawrence's often-banned *Lady Chatterly's Lover*? For beautiful writing and sizzling sex scenes, we also recommend *A Concise Chinese-English Dictionary for Lovers* by Xiaolu Guo. It's about a Chinese woman who moves to London to learn English, and, thanks to an Englishman, learns much, much more.

For those of you who get secretly (or not so secretly) turned on by the thought of the fairer sex, look out for *Virgin Territory*, a collection of essays written by women about their first-time erotic experience with another woman. This out-of-print anthology was compiled by Shar Rednour.

Other suggestions: *Bared to You* by Sylvia Day has the romantic, heavy breathing sex of *Fifty Shades* without the scary S&M. Then again, if you like the scary S&M, author Anne Rice has reawakened her erotic fantasy trilogy of sex slave novels (first published in the 1980s under the pseudonym of A.N. Roquelaure). The trilogy starts with *The Claiming of Sleeping Beauty* in which the Prince awakens Beauty from her 100-year sleep with much more than a simple kiss.

And for the romantics out there, here's an excerpt of Prevention.com's recommendations:

- *A Groom Of One's Own* by Maya Rodale. Why would an upstanding duke consider jilting his duchess bride for a newspaper writer? One word: Passion. A lot of it.
- *Lust In The Library* by Amelia Fayer. "This novella is a great introduction to erotica," says Rodale. Plus, the tagline is hilarious: "Some like it hot. Some like it in the reference section."
- *Aqua Erotica* by Mary Anne Mohanraj. This page-turner explores sexual satisfaction beneath the waves.
- *Seducing Sarah (The Madame X School of Sex)* by Jinx Jamison. For anyone who has wanted to break free from their boring day-to-day life (and who hasn't?), here's your chance to live vicariously through a paralegal who enrolls in sex school—trading mundane meetings for ménage seminars.
- *Lady Sophie's Lover* by Lisa Kleypas. "You cannot go wrong with a Lisa Kleypas novel. She has a gift for beautiful, passionate writing—especially the love scenes," says Rodale.
- *The Dom of My Dreams: A BDSM (bondage & discipline; sadism and masochism) novel*, by M.F. Sinclair. They say never mix business with pleasure, but when a publicist takes on a hot new writer, all the rules go out the window.

Source: www.prevention.com

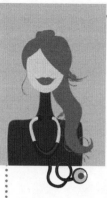

What Your Doctor Can Do

— *Dr. Mary and Dr. Clinton*

Certainly, you can consider a visit to your doctor to talk about your options for a medicinal fix. When I graduated from medical school 15 years ago, I strongly encouraged every woman in my practice to start hormone replacement therapy (HRT) and stay on it forever. We thought that HRT would keep women's hair and nails young and strong. We expected it to reduce rates of cancer, heart disease, memory loss and osteoporosis. Of course, we also counseled that women taking HRT would see a decrease in vasomotor instability, the hot flashes and night sweats that can range from annoying to unbearable during the menopausal transition.

Now, doctors are singing a different tune. Many large and small trials have looked at all kinds of purported risks and benefits of HRT. They conclude that it's probably reasonable to restrict the widespread use of HRT in postmenopausal women. Research is limited by the size and duration of the studies, as well as by the product the researchers decided to use. We don't know, for example, if an outcome seen in a small study is repeatable in a different part of the country, with different researchers, using slightly different techniques, and fewer or more study subjects. It is also unlikely that one study outcome utilizing one type of supplement can be broadly applied to every woman taking a similar product. Tiny

molecular changes can make a big difference in the ability of a molecule to bind with or stimulate a receptor. Results from one study simply are not generalizable across a wide range of people, in most cases. Regarding HRT, as is the case with many chronic conditions, we have to rely on thoughtful input from experts in the field until excellent clinical research data is obtained.

For example, many patients and clinicians alike rely on results from the Women's Health Initiative, commonly referred to as WHI. Started in 1991, WHI followed 161,808 healthy women, and consisted of a set of clinical trials and an observational study. Women who were 65 years or older were placed on either estrogen-alone or estrogen-plus-progestin and followed for 15 years. Based on WHI, we can say that compared with placebo, estrogen-plus-progestin increased the rate of heart attack, stroke, blood clots and breast cancer, and reduced the risk of colorectal cancer. Women on this form of supplementation experienced fewer fractures, but received no benefit against mild cognitive impairment and actually saw an increased risk of dementia. In the estrogen-alone portion of the study, women saw no difference for heart attack, an increased risk of stroke and blood clots, an uncertain effect for breast cancer, no difference in risk for colorectal

cancer, and a reduced risk for fracture compared to women who didn't take HRT.

While this study population is huge, and the duration of the study was very long, and I'm sure very expensive, the premise is all wrong. In real life, a doctor would never start an asymptomatic woman over 65 on hormone replacement therapy. While some experts think the data are generalizable to the general population, others argue that a women who is just beginning her menopausal transition may experience a different set of risks, or quite possibly no risk at all, particularly if HRT is initiated early and consistently administered shortly after the natural withdrawal of estrogen. Some argue that the particular supplemental product that they just happen to sell is without sinister side effects or serious long-term consequences. We just don't know.

For these reasons, HRT is recommended in women who are experiencing vasomotor instability, such as hot flashes and night sweats, and for vaginal atrophy related to menopause. HRT should only be used for osteoporosis protection when a woman does not tolerate the other alternatives.

If you decide to initiate HRT, be careful about the administration of serum tests or saliva tests to measure the levels. These tests are often inaccurate and there is wide variability in the results and lack of effective standardization. This means that your results may not be reliable or reproducible from test to test. Again, we just don't know what your estrogen, progestin and testosterone levels were when you were premenopausal and feeling great. Therefore, we don't know if you are going to need a just a little or a whole lot of estrogen to reach your baseline. The best menopausal clinician will listen to their patient, determine their symptoms, and treat with a product that is formulated to manage their complaints. Then, after several months on therapy, they should have another long visit together to determine if the specific complaints are better.

Don't forget that hormones may not be the source of your problems. Changes in sex drive, appetite or hair loss can represent any number of metabolic derangements, not just hormone deficiencies. Check with your doctor, but keep an open mind to the vast number of possible disorders that could be contributing to your physical complaints.

Testosterone

That said, there is some proven benefits to the addition of HRT, specifically for sexual function. Women supplemented with estrogen and estrogen with progestin have improved responsiveness in multiple laboratory settings, using pornographic materials as the stimulant. Again, these studies are not without their own limitations. While pornographic materials may be valuable in a research setting, a typical bedroom or relationship doesn't really look like a glossy magazine.

Similarly, researchers have more recently found that supplementation with low doses of testosterone further enhance female sexual response to pornographic materials. Testosterone was never thought to be a big deal in women's sexuality. Levels of testosterone in women's blood is only 10 percent the level found in men, but it is thought to play an important role in sexual desire and assertiveness in premenopausal women. Some hormone specialists think that the charming, acquiescing little old lady result is largely because she is devoid of the testosterone. With the withdrawal of testosterone, it's thought

that women not only lose some of their sexual desire, but also some of their assertiveness. Testosterone is produced in the ovary, and although blood levels decline dramatically after menopause, women experience slow declines over their adulthood so that blood levels of testosterone in a woman in her forties are half the levels that a woman enjoys in her twenties.

Until recently, the only data on testosterone supplementation and sexual desire was from the 1960's using rats as subjects. The study suggested that there is increased desire with supplementation. While the fact that a very poorly designed rat study is somehow extrapolated to the human female is vaguely insulting to me, that was the state of medical research on women back then. In any case, more recent data has shown that women supplemented with testosterone in addition to estrogen/progestin experience a better response to sexual stimuli. In a study published in 1995 in Maturitas, 32 postmenopausal women were treated with estrogen or estrogen/progestin combined with testosterone. Both groups experienced improvement in sexual desire, but the testosterone treated group experienced increased sexual desire over their estrogen-only counterparts. Other studies support these initial findings.

While the data is provocative and worth thoughtful consideration, there are serious side effects to administering any hormone supplementation. In addition to the side effects elucidated by WHI regarding estrogen and progestin, excess testosterone supplementation can cause acne, facial hair growth, changes in the quality of the voice and clitoral enlargement. Administration should probably be transdermal, to decrease the effect of liver breakdown on the product. It should be noted that most oral HRT

is converted to estrogen as it passes through the liver, which makes a patch or crème a smart approach to delivering hormones in their active state. Hormone transport through the liver also results in decreased production of sex hormone binding globulin. Sex hormone binding globulins are produced by the liver to bind excess sex hormones and help to stabilize the levels of sex hormones. The combination of increased hormones and decreased production of binding proteins sharply increases the sex hormone levels in the blood. In a study at University Hospitals of Cleveland, over half of the 64 women who tried testosterone patches reported a substantial improvement in their sexual desire, resulting in four to five additional "satisfying" sexual episodes per month.

Food & Estrogen

Balancing your hormones often simply requires a balancing of your diet. When you streamline your diet by removing animal proteins and fats in favor of healthy plant-based nutrition, you reduce your exposure to estrogen and other harmful chemicals present in these foods. In one Harvard study, women eating a plant-based diet saw a reduction in estrogen levels in the blood by 40 percent in just a few short weeks. Reducing excessive estrogen stimulation will allow existing progestin and testosterone, previously crowded out by the excess estrogen, to stimulate their receptors and bring a woman into perfect hormonal balance. Your doctor may have some great advice for hormonal manipulation, but the key to healthy hormonal balance lies in a balanced diet. Similarly, pills like Viagra increase blood flow to the genitals, but a healthy diet is

Continued...

like super-Viagra, allowing unobstructed, healthy blood flow to the genitals and improving mood and energy so that you, gorgeous girl, have all the desire you will ever need.

WHAT IS IT?

Finally, be sure to check the origin of your pharmaceuticals. The estrogen supplement Premarin is made from the urine of pregnant mares, leading to significant animal suffering and some very negative outcomes in the offspring of these horses (most are killed and sold as horsemeat in Europe and Japan; the lucky ones are adopted). Be sure to find a cruelty-free HRT product, if you determine that you need a product at all.

What about "natural" alternatives? There are many of them, including shatavra (derived from wild asparagus, its Sanscrit name means "she who possesses 100 husbands"), maca (considered a "passion" plant native to Peru), and damiana (an aphrodisiac made from a Mexican shrub). How well these products work is unclear. The industry is unregulated, and there are hardly any clinical trials. One exception is the botanical product called Zestra. A very small study reported in the January 2003 issue of Journal of Sex and Marital Therapy found that this oil, which contains borage-seed and evening-primrose oils plus angelica and coleus extracts, was more effective than a placebo for enhancing arousal when applied to the genitals. Often, mint extract is used in products that increase arousal and pleasure. Some people find that it's helpful, while others say it's uncomfortable or even burns. K-Y Intense claims that 70 percent of women surveyed agreed that they experienced increased arousal, satisfaction and pleasure, but these results are not published in the medical literature.

Lubricate!

Many patients have complained to me about pain, especially at the initiation of sex. Of course, a little more foreplay is always a fun idea, but a little extra lubrication can help things along. I used to recommend using Astroglide, which has been the best product on the market for sexual lubrication for years. Plus it has the funniest name. Increasingly, though, I think it is a good idea to avoid the use of mineral oils; there are many terrific organic lubricants available at your health food store or through online catalogs. Many of my patients like Aqua Lube and Emerita, which are natural lubricants made primarily from glycerin. You can also create your own preferred viscosity by combining several different oils.

While some women want lubrication for enhancing sexual function, some women also experience a more general vaginal dryness that is bothersome after menopause. Some women respond very well to Premarin vaginal creme, applied using an applicator inside the vaginal vault just two or three times a week. For those of you who love animals and don't want to contribute to animal suffering from the production of this particular pharmaceutical, consider using an applicator to simply apply a moisturizing oil. Moisturizing oils relieve vaginal dryness without the use of hormones, and my patients report a similar response of the tissues to moisturizing, with or without the concomitant use of hormones in the moisturizing creme. It's easy to pick up an applicator at the drugstore, in the same section where you can purchase over the counter antifungal products for vaginal yeast infections. For lubrication and general moisturizing, I recommend walnut oil. Walnuts are crazy high in omega-3 fats, which support elastic, supple tissues. A little walnut oil applied intravaginally works very well to support healthy tissues and waning lubrication. I would avoid oils that have a high concentration of omega-6 fatty acids, since these fats are less healthy than omega-3 fats. Oils that are higher in healthy fats include olive oil, walnut oil and canola oil. Flaxseed oil has the highest concentration of omega-3 fats of all the refined oils. Corn, peanut, safflower, sesame and sunflower oil are the highest in omega-6 fats. Vaginal mucosa is thin and permeable, so anything you put in your vagina is highly likely to get into your bloodstream, at least in small amounts. Also, anything you put in your vagina is getting very close to a lot of other important organs, like your ovaries and your colon. It is also getting very close to important organs on your partner, like his testicles and prostate. Make sure that you choose a healthy, organic moisturizer and personal lubricant, as the safest alternative for you and your partner. Choose a few oils from your local health food store and have some fun experimenting with them. Find the one that works best for you and your specific needs.

Here is a table that may be helpful to you as you go about selecting some refined oils for personal lubrication purposes:

Type of Oil	Omega-3	Omega-6	Monounsaturated Fat	Saturated Fat
Flaxsseed	57	16	18	9
Rapeseed	10	22	62	6
Soybean	7	54	24	15
Walnut	5	51	28	16
Olive (extra virgin)	1	8	77	14
Corn	1	61	25	13
Peanut	0	33	49	18
Safflower	0	77	13	10
Sesame	0	41	46	13
Sunflower	0	69	20	11

You're in the Mood

Also give some consideration to the angle of entry. I'm talking about excessive pelvic tilting, resulting in an extreme angle of entry that creates undue pressure on the perineum, the area between and vagina and anus. Try to relax your pelvis a bit in anticipation of entry, straightening the arch in your back, and see if that reduces some of the initial discomfort. Small positional changes combined with a suitable lubricant, may go a long way toward restoring your sexual pleasure.

Chronic pain, urinary problems, and fatigue can all decrease your interest in sex, as can medications such as antidepressants, antihistamines, and blood pressure drugs. Again, your plant-based diet improves your mood, reduces your risk for blood pressure, and eases allergies, making some or all of these medications unnecessary. As you ease into a healthy diet, you should see dramatic reductions in your need for medications to manage multiple, chronic medical conditions.

Ditch the Kids

Once you figure out what's right for you, consider sending the kids to their friend's house, and preparing a little private romantic dinner for you and your baby daddy. Maybe some candles could be burning, why not? I think I'm hearing a little Michael Bublé in the background. There's the flesh and blood in front of you that initially turned your head so long ago, and there's the heart and soul that really made you fall in love forever. Sit down and enjoy some time talking and listening, sharing your history and looking forward to the future. Then go to bed and make love. And for the night after that, schedule a rubdown to further increase the release of oxytocin, and surprise your husband again.

A great friend is important in a partner, but great sex, well, great sex matters too. The combination of the shortest time from stimulation to orgasm and a plant-based diet just might mean that a woman in their forties and fifties can actually be experiencing the best sex of her life. All these kids have no idea what they can look forward to!

SPICE UP YOUR SKIN

Antioxidants called carotenoids give vegetables like carrots and sweet potatoes their color, and researchers found that they also lend a pleasant glow to our skin. When participants were shown pictures of people tanned by the sun and others who ate lots of carotenoids, they thought the veggie eaters were more attractive than the tanners. The golden hue in the skin of people eating a carotenoid-rich diet beat out the look of suntan, according to studies from the University of Nottingham. The researchers think that the carotenoid-hued skin of healthy dieters is enticing because it suggests a healthy partner. Carotenoids may attract mates, but they also give the immune system a boost and may even help slow the appearance of aging.

So, want to get the glowing skin for yourself? Carotenoids are found in winter vegetables like kale, collard greens and sweet potatoes. Apricots, mangoes and tomatoes can also contribute to healthy looking skin. Or spice up your meal with cayenne or chili pepper, both of which contain carotenoids. Don't forget about carrots and squash too.

HEALTHY DIET — HEALTHY SKIN

Have you ever noticed how women who follow a plant-based diet have such gorgeous skin? Another consideration in waning sexual response is the aging of the skin. While no formal studies have been undertaken, many companies are developing products that are designed specifically for the vagina, clitoris and nipples. This year, LELO plans to offer 24 new products, including nipple masks, nipple spray, and "anti-aging and cellular renewal cream" for the vagina, clitoris, nipples and the skin around the inner thighs. Donna Faro, director of sales and marketing for LELO, said, "We have studied the skin, and we understand what's lacking in areas of a woman as she ages."

Anyone interested in the maintenance of healthy skin should start with a healthy diet. Before you decide to throw a lot of your hard-earned dollars toward expensive topical preparations, modify your diet to include plants, whole grains and beans. These foods are naturally rich in the healthy omega-3 fats that make skin supple, and the micronutrients that lead to a glowing complexion.

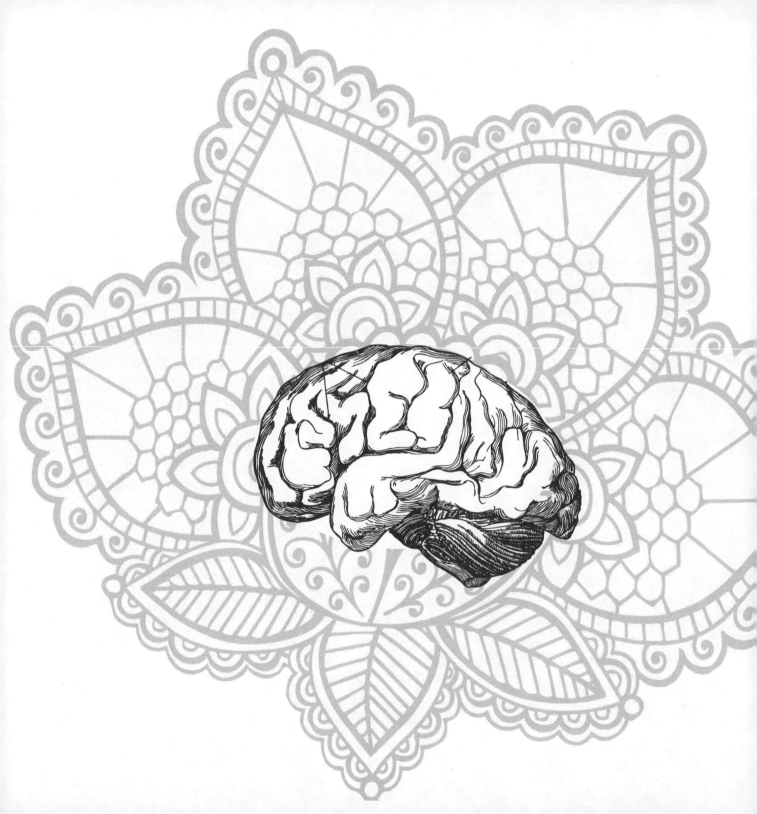

Your Brain on Fat
— Dr. Clinton —

Scientists in California have great new information on the effect of a high-fat diet on brain function, but it is important to understand what happens to dietary fat after it is consumed. Excess fat, of course, is put into storage for later use. There is a physiologic level of healthy fat that we all need to support cellular function. Most of this essential fat is used to build cellular membranes, the delicate bi-layer of fatty acids that separate the insides of cells from the extracellular fluid. This is where the deposition of healthy fats—and I am talking omega-3 fats—makes all the difference in the health of your brain and in your metabolic rate.

The best way to think about your dietary fats is to classify them as omega-3 and omega-6. These fatty acids are different based on their molecular structure. The side chains present on omega-6 fatty acids render the molecule very stiff and stable, while the side chains on omega-3 fatty acids result in a less stable, but highly flexible molecule. The food choices in the Standard American Diet heavily favor a high concentration of omega-6 fatty acids and those are linked to all kinds of negative health outcomes.

In countries with less disease and healthier plant-based diets, the ratio of omega-6 to omega-3 fats is 3:1. In our meat-eating country, ordinary people have ratios of at least 15:1, but sometimes as high as 20:1 or even 25:1. A healthier, lower ratio of omega-6 to omega-3 is associated with less cardiovascular disease, less chronic disease, better health in general and a higher functioning brain as you age.

Why is omega-3 so much better for you than omega-6? Well, the membranes in your body cells are made up of a phospholipid bi-layer, which is basically two layers of fats that tuck their hydrophobic (water-fearing) tails toward each other and put their hydrophilic (water-loving) heads toward the outside of the cell. This is where the omega-3 fatty acids in a plant-based diet work their magic.

When the cellular membranes contain a high concentration of omega-3 fats, the membranes are squishy and flexible. Two remarkable things happen when the cell membranes are squishy and flexible. First, it's easier for the vital proteins that are created outside the cell to cross the phospholipid cellular membrane and get into the cell's interior. The cell membranes effectively twist and bend to allow the protein to transport through. In short, proteins and other important cellular products are able to be in the right place at the right time and that ensures the health and integrity of cellular function throughout the entire body. This is important in multiple tissues, but it's critically important in the aging human brain.

In contrast, when people eat a diet high in animal products, they effectively concentrate their fat sources with omega-6 fats, which create cell walls that are inflexible and stiff. When the cellular membrane is too stiff, these transport proteins have quite a bit of trouble. The extracellular protein attempting transport can get stuck in the membrane or break off as it tries to enter the cell. Vital proteins are able to wiggle and bend and end up getting stuck in the cell membrane.

The second remarkable thing that happens when a cell wall is flexible and squishy is that the cell wall is also rendered very leaky. Leaky cell walls result in more sodium and potassium moving in and out of the cell. This requires more hard work from the sodium-potassium pumps to maintain appropriate levels of critical electrolytes in these environments. For you, that means that each individual cell is working harder to keep basic cellular environments together. That, my dear friend, means an increased metabolic rate for the healthy eater consuming a high concentration of omega-3 fatty acid. As each cell works harder to maintain the environment, the entire system burns more energy and the healthy whole-foods, plant-based eater is suddenly finding it much easier to lose weight.

Getting great levels of omega-3 fats is easy when you are following a plant-based diet. Plant and marine foods are good sources of omega-3 fats. In general, the higher the fat content of the plant food you are eating, the higher the level of omega-3 fats in the plant.

That doesn't mean that the plant-based eater needs to focus on getting high fat plants like avocado and nuts in their diet everyday. Just by eating a wide variety of plants and removing the animal products, the ratio of fats normalizes.

When you are looking for healthy fats, just look to plant-based foods. Enjoy a healthy, balanced diet with plenty of fresh fruits and vegetables and you'll have the perfect ratio of fats to thrive.

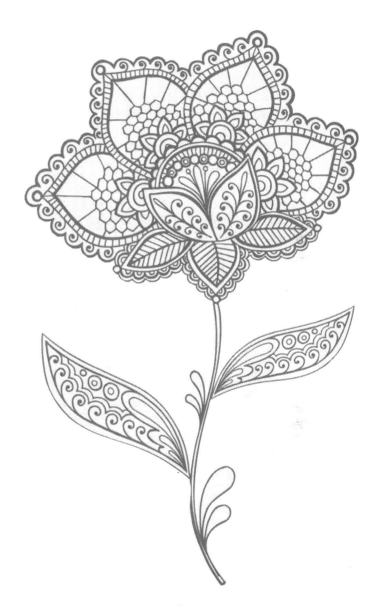

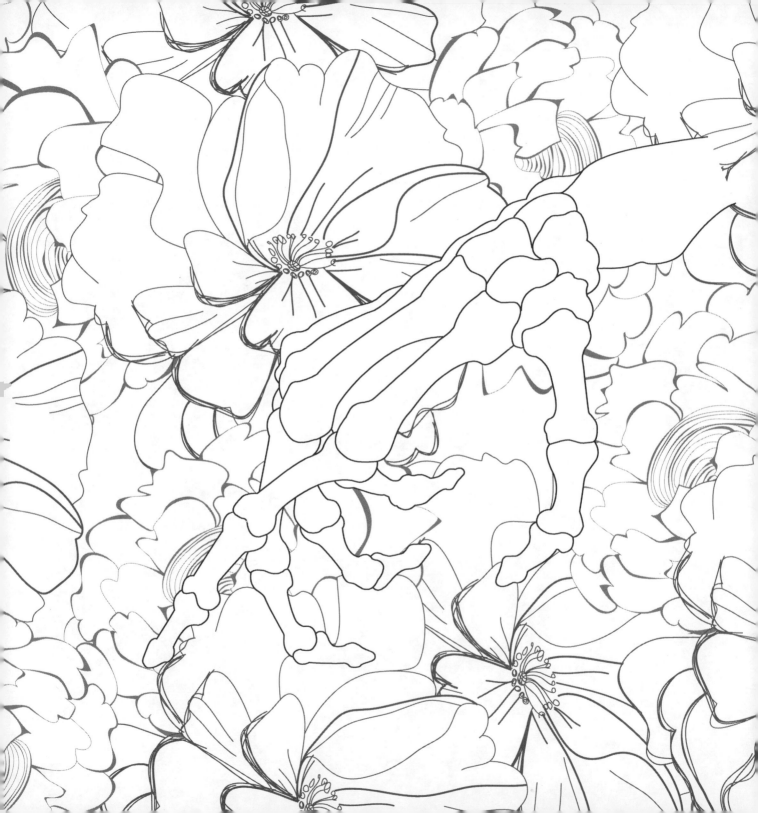

Feeding Your Bones
— Dr. Clinton —

Bone is made up of proteins that bind to each other, creating strong cross links that support the weight of the other structures in the body, like muscles and organs. There are two types of bone in the human skeleton: Trabecular bone is found in the inside of bones. When it's healthy, it looks like very good Swiss cheese, or like the steel structure of a skyscraper in the process of being built. The outer layer of bone, the cortex, is made up of cortical bone. Cortical bone is thicker and denser, and functions like a strong outer protective shell for the inner latticework.

What keeps bones strong and healthy, and why do some of us suffer from bone weakness? It all has to do with bone turnover, and that's a subject keenly interesting to Dr. David Dempster. He is a bone scientist who has spent 40 years studying bone turnover at Cornell University in upstate New York.

Imagine that you just initiated a running program, and that you've unfortunately developed micro-fractures in your tibia, commonly referred to as shin splints. I'm going to explain what happens at the cellular level so that you can connect the boring science to the more exciting implications for diet. So here goes! Your body releases molecules that are known as local inflammatory mediators—essentially cells that, like an ambulance, arrive at sites of inflammation to promote healing, cells such as interleukin-1 and tumor necrosis factor. These mediators activate the osteogenic precursor cells—cells that come from bone-forming tissue. These cells then morph into osteoclasts, which are cells that clean up and sweep away dirty, old bone. The osteoclasts swing into action and clean the bone. After the osteoclasts finish their work, they leave behind a resorptive pit, or a space that's ready to fill in with fresh new bone. Osteoblasts—osteogenic precursor cells that have morphed into building cells—go to the site of the resorptive pit and fill it in with fresh, new bone. The process of building a new bony surface takes only four to six weeks. Mineralizing that site with calcium and phosphorus to harden and strengthen the site takes another several weeks.

In a woman's premenopausal years, the osteoclastic and osteoblastic functions are beautifully balanced —when old, dirty bone is identified, it is cleaned up and promptly replaced with fresh healthy bone. After estrogen levels decline, however, the osteoclast function—the cells that clean up and sweep away dirty old bone—increases dramatically, but the osteoblast bone-building activities get overwhelmed by bone resorption. There are just not enough osteoblast precursor cells to go around. This results in an overall loss of bone in the postmenopausal woman, particularly in the first three years of menopause.

Bones are remarkably responsive, dynamic structures. Trabecular bone, the inner structure of most bones, turns over at a rate of 22 percent per year. Cortical bone, that outer hard surface of bones, turns over at a rate of only 3 percent per year. When a woman undergoes menopause, however, bone turnover increases by 8 percent for the first three years after the transition, resulting in a remarkably rapid loss of bone early in the menopausal transition.

Protecting the bone through healthy exercise and diet becomes critical during this phase of life. According to Dr. Bonny Specker, the world thought leader on exercise and bone health, the very best exercise for bone building is tennis. There's plenty of acceleration and rapid deceleration (running and stopping), weighted rotation (swinging the racket) and weight-bearing exercise (jumping) for the entire skeleton. Increasingly, scientists are looking not only at the distance or duration of exercise, but at the acceleration and deceleration that occurs during the exercise. Stopping and starting, like running or basketball may have more skeletal benefits than exercising exclusively with yoga or walking.

Mix It Up

If you aren't a tennis player, identify a number of different activities you do like to do. Biking is great, but bikers are prone to osteoporosis of the mid-spine due to lack of use. Walking is great too, but it doesn't work the shoulder girdle and upper spine very well. Combining a few different activities will benefit your entire body's skeleton and muscle system. This is why so many excellent personal trainers recommend you do a wide range of activities through cross training.

Keep Calcium in Your Bones

Remember Dr. Dempster? Turns out he wrote the paper on nutrition and osteoporosis

ON THE LIGHT SIDE ...

I encourage my patients to find natural, whole food sources for all of their nutrition needs. I was counseling a skinny little old lady about getting vitamin D from the sun. Just one 15-minute exposure of the chest and arms to direct sunlight converts enough cholesterol in the skin to vitamin D for a whole week of healthy cellular metabolism. I jokingly suggested she put on her tube top and head out to the garden. "Oh, Dr. Mary", she said, "I haven't had a tube top on in five years."

She's 85.

—DR. MARY

way back in the 1980s. He studied the function of osteoclasts in great detail. When osteoclasts get ready to sweep away bone, they adhere themselves to the surface of the bone. The osteoclast then creates a pocket of highly acidic fluid between itself and the bone. It is in this highly acidic environment that the osteoclast works to sweep away damaged bone. Dr. Dempster's laboratory work showed that when the acidity of the microenvironment rose even slightly, the osteoclasts went crazy with increased activity. The acidic microenvironment theoretically makes their job of creating a highly acidic pocket much easier. They are able to work faster to absorb and sweep away bone.

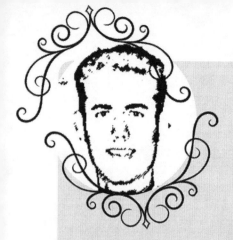

THE BEST THING YOU CAN DO FOR YOUR BONES?

MOVE! A LOT!

BY DR. STEPHAN ESSER, MD

FOUNDER OF THE ESSER FOUNDATION

"These boots were meant for walking" . . . or so the classic song goes. The lyrics are spot on. Not only the boots though, your whole body is meant for walking . . . and swimming, jumping, dancing, biking, spinning and so much more. You were meant to be active every day, everywhere. The science is clear, along with health-promoting food, regular physical activity is the most powerful thing you can do to look and feel younger, achieve ideal weight, prevent disease, keep your bones strong, promote function and maintain the highest quality of life possible.

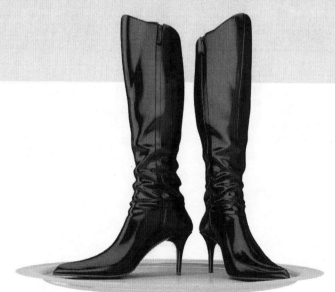

The acidic microenvironment purportedly created by a diet rich in animal proteins theoretically results in accelerated osteoclastic function, according to Dr. Dempster's research. Remember hearing that meat doesn't really digest; it just rots in your gut? When a woman eats a diet rich in animal proteins, this results in a prolonged acidic environment in the gut. The increased gut acidity results in increased acidity in the blood.

The body's chemistry becomes vital when talking about bones, but it's another one of those subjects that gets complicated fast. Think about it like this: When my mom gets a sour stomach, she often chews a calcium carbonate tablet for instant acid indigestion relief, under the trade name of Tums. This is exactly what the body is doing when it is going to the bone for calcium salts in an effort to neutralize the acidity created by animal foods. But how do animal foods create acid?

In the digestion process of animal proteins, the proteins must undergo extensive methylation and hydroxylation. These chemical processes result in the creation of acids. The body rids itself of these excess acids by peeing them out in the urine. But in order to neutralize the acidity of the urine, the body grabs extra calcium from the bones and that's peed out too—in the same way my mom neutralizes her excess acidity by taking a Tums. The advantage vegans hold is that plants do not create an acid environment in the body and, therefore, the body isn't stimulated to leach calcium from the bones to neutralize the acid.

Recent studies, however, have argued that urinary acidification/calcification associated with a high protein diet may not be accurate. These researchers gave women very large doses of animal proteins combined with a large dose of calcium that was radioactively tagged, so they could see where the calcium ended up. They noted that the radioactively tagged calcium ended up in the blood serum and urine after women consumed a large amount of protein. The researchers concluded that the calcium in the urine of women consuming a high protein diet actually originates from the food they are eating, not from their own bones. The research also suggests that a high protein diet leads to increased calcium absorption— that is the intestines of omnivores more readily absorb calcium from food.

This study seems to raise more questions than it answers. If a high protein diet is consumed with high concentrations of calcium, then the body will not have to look to the skeletal system for additional calcium to handle the increased urinary acidity. However, if the woman's diet is deficient in calcium, as is true in Western diets, then the body will naturally have to look to the skeleton as a source of calcium. Further study in this area, with a more realistic combination of a high protein diet with low calcium ingestion, might provide more insightful on how diet affects skeletal health.

Not all animal proteins are created equal, according to research by Dr. T Colin Campbell and Boston nutrition expert Dr. Beth Dawson-Hughes. Meats and processed dairy products such as hard cheeses generate acid

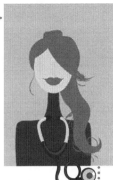

What Your Doctor Can Do *—Dr. Clinton*

While the US government and medical associations recommend 1200 to 1800 mg of calcium per day, the World Health Organization and many foreign countries recommend about 500 mg per day. A large study published in the spring of 2010 showed that women supplementing with calcium tablets have an increased risk of death due to heart attack and stroke. Women were especially at risk if they were already eating large sources of calcium in their diet and supplementing with a concentrated calcium supplement. At this point, I would recommend that women get at least 500 mg of calcium from healthy dietary sources, including whole grains, beans, plant milk and green leafy vegetables, while dramatically limiting their exposure to animal proteins. If their diets are crummy, they should work on their diets, and supplement their calcium to at least 500 mg daily until their diets are improved.

66 DID YOU KNOW?

That almond milk has nearly twice the calcium of a glass of cow's milk? One cup of almond milk contains 459 milligrams of calcium compared to 276 milligrams of calcium in a cup of cow's milk. So you get the calcium you need without the saturated fat, cholesterol, casein, gluten and MSG. Most almond milk products are also fortified with Vitamin D and E.

CALCIUM: WHERE OH WHERE CAN IT BE?

Adding high calcium plant foods to your regular diet will boost your calcium intake and leave you with a strong, powerful skeleton. Here are just a few of the high calcium foods that you can rely on as you transition to a plant-based diet. When you start to worry about absorption or bioavailability, remember that giraffes, zebras, horses and deer maintain their graceful appearance and perfect skeletons on plants, just plants, with no dairy after they are weaned from their mommas. Look at the impressive calcium content of greens and seeds. No wonder the gals in the Women's Health Initiative who ate just one salad a week saw a 40 percent reduction in fractures over their salad-avoiding counterparts.

These measurements were obtained from 3.5 ounce serving sizes of these foods.

Almonds 234 mg

Amaranth 267 mg

Apricots (dried) 67 mg

Artichokes 51 mg

Beans (can: pinto, black) 135 mg

Beet greens (cooked) 99 mg

Bran 70 mg

Buckwheat 114 mg

Cabbage (raw) 49 mg

Chickpeas (garbanzos) 150 mg

Collards (raw leaves) 250 mg

Figs (dried) 126 mg

Hazelnuts 209 mg

Kale (raw leaves) 249 mg

Kale (cooked leaves) 187 mg

Leeks 52 mg

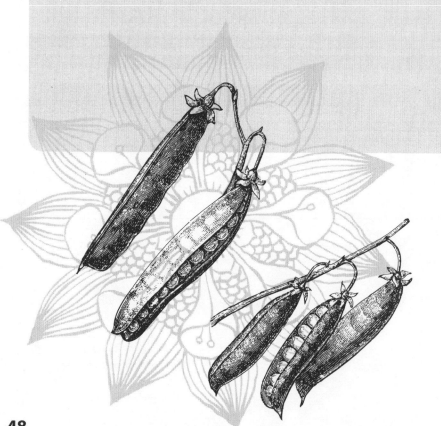

Lettuce (dark green) 68 mg

Molasses (dark-213 cal.) 684 mg

Mustard Greens (raw) 183 mg

Olives 61 mg

Oranges (Florida) 43 mg

Parsley 203 mg

Peanuts (roasted & salted) 74 mg

Peas (boiled) 56 mg

Pistachio Nuts 131 mg

Raisins 62 mg

Soybeans 60 mg

Tofu 128 mg

Spinach (raw) 93 mg

Sunflower Seeds 120 mg

Turnip Greens (raw) 246 mg

Water Cress 151 mg

DO YOU HAVE A VITAMIN D DEFICIT?
MAYBE IT'S BECAUSE YOU'RE DRINKING DAIRY ...

How many of you are taking a vitamin D supplement? This is the first time that a nutritional supplement has caught the attention of the medical community with such fervor since I began my practice. And I admit, the initial evaluation of the material is alluring. Fights colon cancer, lowers risk of depression, all kinds of stuff. Sounds a lot like the benefits I get from the veg diet I try to follow.

Dr. Beth Dawson-Hughes did the research that led to the government increasing the recommended daily allowance of Vitamin D. She brought 5,000 volunteers to her office and measured their blood levels of vitamin D. She found that high levels of activated vitamin D were associated with lower rates of disease. Those results got generalized to any and all levels of vitamin D, but physicians are just not seeing the benefit of supplementing vitamin D like we thought we would based on the initial data.

What gives? We haven't looked at why people off the street would walk into Beth's office with a high level of activated vitamin D. Vitamin D, as you probably know, is available in food supplements, bones of other animals, and is made from the cholesterol in your skin with exposure to the sun. Vitamin D then travels to the kidneys to undergo activation, so it can go to the gut and collect tiny pieces of calcium from your healthy diet. Activated vitamin D lives for that purpose, to find tiny particles of calcium from your food. Folks who get their calcium in small amounts through beans, greens and whole grains have lots of activated vitamin D in super-charged mode, looking for that special mineral and scooping it up.

When you drink a big glass of milk or take a supplement, your body gets a mega-dose of calcium. A ton of calcium. Then your gut tells your kidneys, don't make any more activated vitamin D. We don't need to go looking for calcium; we have a ton of the stuff. And your kidneys do what they are told. So people who ingest the highest amount of dairy have the lowest levels of activated vitamin D. Activated vitamin D is quite simply a measure of a person's exposure to dairy. And because dairy has high levels of insulin-like growth factor, fats and calories—all of which grows tumors like crazy—these folks have higher levels of all the chronic diseases like cancer, heart disease, obesity and diabetes.

Which is why the dairy-loving USA has epidemic levels of activated vitamin D deficiency, and why other countries don't suffer like we do. The government recommends between 1,200 to 1,800 mg of calcium per day. The World Health Organization and many other countries recommend 500 mg per day. I recently read that these differences in recommendations are due to different levels of vitamin D deficiency. Maybe it has more to do with our source of dietary calcium.

Excerpted from Dr. Mary's blog, http://drmarymd.com

during their digestion. Liquid milk, however, is alkaline in the body, and does not promote urinary acidification and calcification like other dairy products. You still might want to avoid liquid milk for other reasons, but more on that later. It is not reasonable to issue a blanket warning that all animal proteins are harmful to your bones.

Perhaps the most reassuring bit of data arose from a study of Buddhist nuns, women who were vegans for most or all of their lives. The bone density of these nuns was measured and compared to the bone density of ordinary women. It turns out that the nuns had clinically equivalent bone mineral density to women who drank cow's milk and consumed nearly twice as much calcium in their daily diet.

To suggest that dairy products aren't the healthiest source of dietary calcium and protein is almost unpatriotic here in the United States. We Americans grew up as little girls with milk on our cereal at breakfast, a carton of milk on the corner of our lunch tray and a glass of milk at the corner of our placemat at dinner. Copious scientific data have made it clear that we have healthier, safer protein and calcium sources in beans and whole grains, without the inflammation and acidification risks associated with animal proteins. While plenty of government programs subsidize meat and dairy, women have to recognize that the government is often slow to respond to new information. Women seeking optimal health should focus on the identification of plant sources of calcium like green leafy vegetables, whole grains and beans.

Getting to Know Your Skeleton

You can ask your doctor to perform a bone density test to determine the density of your skeleton. Bone density can be measured by ultrasound, plain x-ray or a quantitative CT scanning of the vertebrae (back) or femur (thigh) bone, but the most common method is the use of bone densitometry. The technology is readily available everywhere, and you don't even have to undress to undergo the testing. You can simply lie down on the examination table while the machine records your bone density in just a few moments. The radiation exposure is equivalent to a day in the sun. Most advisory boards recommend starting bone density measurements at 65 years old, repeating them as often as necessary based on the bone density measurement, risk for developing osteoporosis and risks for fracture. For example, the need for treatment or frequency of testing is different for a healthy gal who has low bone density, compared to a gal who doesn't eat properly, smokes, takes multiple medications and who is at risk of falling because of limited vision. Your doctor should carefully balance all of the risks and benefits of therapy before initiating any medical management. You can also use risk calculators available to your doctor through the National Osteoporosis Foundation to help determine your risk of fracture more accurately.

SHOULD YOU WORRY ABOUT VITAMINS AND MINERALS?

The USDA website has a very comprehensive listing of micronutrients in foods. When I first made my dietary switch, I kept my laptop computer open in the kitchen and referred to the site continually while I cooked, until I felt confident that I was getting adequate calcium and protein from beans, rice and vegetables. That's where I learned that one avocado has twelve grams of fiber! But as Dr. Hans Diehl, the founder of the CHIP program and leading nutritional expert says, if you take care of the macro, the micro takes care of itself. If you are choosing healthy sources of protein, fats and carbohydrates, you needn't worry about vitamins and minerals. There is really no need to fret over your calcium, or your protein, or your fiber. If you are eating a plant-based diet with whole foods (not processed), your nutritional status will improve astronomically over the Standard American Diet.

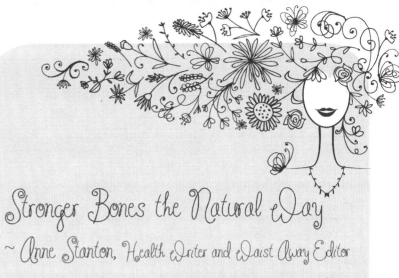

Stronger Bones the Natural Way
~ Anne Stanton, Health Writer and Waist Away Editor

In the summer of 2008, I had a bone density test. At the time I was a 51-year-old, tall, slim and post-menopausal woman. So I guess I was at risk, with bones thinning once you hit menopause. I was also genetically at risk. My grandma, who has a similar build, became very hunched over in old age and shrunk a good three inches before her death at age 92.

So the bone density test was easy—far more comfortable than a mammogram. You just lie down on a table and get sort of wanded by a machine. I felt like a piece of paper in a copy machine. A short time later, my doctor called me in and said my bone mineral density was on the low side. It was almost low enough to qualify as osteopenia or pre-osteoporosis. She was concerned and suggested that I begin taking calcium supplements. And I did.

Well, a year later I became a vegetarian and read that meat products alter the pH of the body to a slightly acidic state. To help bring the body into a stable, neutral pH, the body leaches calcium from the bones. Do you remember that from chemistry? A base in balance with acid equals a nice neutral pH of seven. At the same time, I learned that taking calcium supplements might not be so wise. In fact, it can actually increase the chances for kidney stones (particularly if you don't take them with a meal). My sister, who had just suffered a kidney stone, called it a pain worse than childbirth. So I felt my best bet was to ensure that I ate lots of calcium from vegetable sources such as tofu, spinach and broccoli. I also continued to jog, which I also read is great for your bones.

Three years later, I got another bone density scan. And guess what? Completely normal! I am not kidding. My doctor was happy, too, but told me to continue taking calcium supplements. When I told her that I hadn't been taking them for two years, she was a little aghast. It's a little scary to go against the recommendations of mainstream medicine, but I don't think you can go wrong by eating calcium-rich foods instead of swallowing pills. Since that first bone scan in 2008, I feel further vindicated. Clinical studies are showing that calcium supplements increase the risk of heart attacks, which run in my family, and early death.

What to Do if You're Diagnosed with Osteoporosis

Osteoporosis treatment is reasonable when diet and exercise fails to control bone loss, or when bone loss is complicated with fracture. As women age, the main reasons for loss of independence and transfer to nursing homes are dementia and bone fracture. Preventing fracture, therefore, is a very important part of successful aging. To prevent a fall, do the easy things first. Remove any clutter from the floor and tape down or remove any loose carpets or rugs that may get caught on the edge of a foot and lead to falls. Make sure that if you need a walking aid, you use it regularly. If your doctor thinks you would benefit from using a cane, go ahead and buy a cane to stabilize your posture, and then use it. It'll do you no good propped up against the wall instead of held in your hand.

Long-term treatment with many bone-stabilizing medications is falling under scrutiny recently, since these medications have been linked to atypical fracture in the femur and osteonecrosis of the jaw (bone death caused by poor blood supply). Researchers are concerned that prolonged treatment with osteoporosis medications may result in the suppression of bone turnover until the bone is no longer able to properly heal itself by cleaning up and replacing old, damaged bone. As a result, damaged bone may accumulate, which increases risk for fracture. If you have been treated for many years with osteoporosis medications, it may be time to talk to your doctor.

While there is talk of taking a "drug holiday," where patients stop their osteoporosis medications for a while, there are no scientific studies to support that idea.

When considering a drug holiday, it's important to note that adequate data on fracture risk is collected in just three short years of study in most drug trials. If you are osteoporotic at high risk of fracture because of falls or other chronic disease, it doesn't take long to experience a serious outcome, like fracture and disability, from your osteoporosis. If you have osteoporosis, you are at higher risk for fracture, and given the consequences of fractures, taking prescribed medications makes a lot of sense. The FDA does recommend that potent osteoporosis therapy is limited to three to five years, at which time therapeutic need should be reassessed. There are new medications and alternatives that don't have the same level of risk associated with their administration, and a little subtle change in your medication, in addition to a great, healthy diet and exercise plan, may be just the thing you need.

LITTLE OLD LADIES ARE LITTLE FOR A REASON

—DR. MARY

When I was a brand-new doctor, freshly graduated from medical school and in residency training, my attending physicians taught me that hip fractures could ultimately kill patients. Prevention of hip fracture took precedence over other fractures, and consequently the risks of other fractures were largely ignored. That is, until an Australian study. When the Australians studied over 10,000 women, instead of just several hundred as in previous studies, they were able to show that there are mortality risks with all fractures, even very slight increased risks for fractures of the wrist! Even small limitations, such as the inability to button a blouse after wrist fracture, may lead to an older woman to decide to skip lunch out with her girlfriends and eat some crackers in front of the TV at home. This not only eliminates the brain-stimulating opportunity of pleasant conversation with her gal pals, but also limits her nutritional status. Other elderly women, after suffering from one fracture, often fear falling in the middle of the night when they get up to go to the bathroom. So they decide to stop drinking water after dinner—and that can lead to dehydration, possible dizziness and falling. Exactly what they were trying to prevent!

Consider the little old lady who is hunched forward with a curved spine. She has likely suffered vertebral compression fractures, which are essentially thinning vertebrae bones that have collapsed due to the pressure of maintaining an upright posture. As the vertebrae collapse and her spine rounds, the woman develops an unsightly bulging tummy and flat bottom. Worse, she finds herself staring at the ground eight feet in front of her, unless she bends her knees and rotates her pelvis forward to reposition her upper body in a more normal posture. The new posture puts pressure on her hips and lower back, often leading to low back pain.

More importantly, the curvature of the spine decreases total airflow in the lungs, dramatically decreasing pulmonary function by approximately 10 percent with each fracture. The forward bend also mashes the organs in the abdomen, leading to compression of the stomach and a sense of feeling "full" after just a few bites. And that can mean nutritional deprivation or even slow starvation for the osteoporotic lady.

For these reasons, the National Osteoporosis Foundation encourages doctors to prevent a first fracture. The biggest indicator that a patient will sustain a fracture is the presence of an existing fracture. By asking doctors to identify and treat the patients at highest risk for fracture and preventing a first fracture, the doctor has a much higher chance of successfully keeping her patient healthy and independent into their advanced age. Waiting to start an intervention after a woman is already suffering with a curved spine is not the best approach to managing osteoporosis.

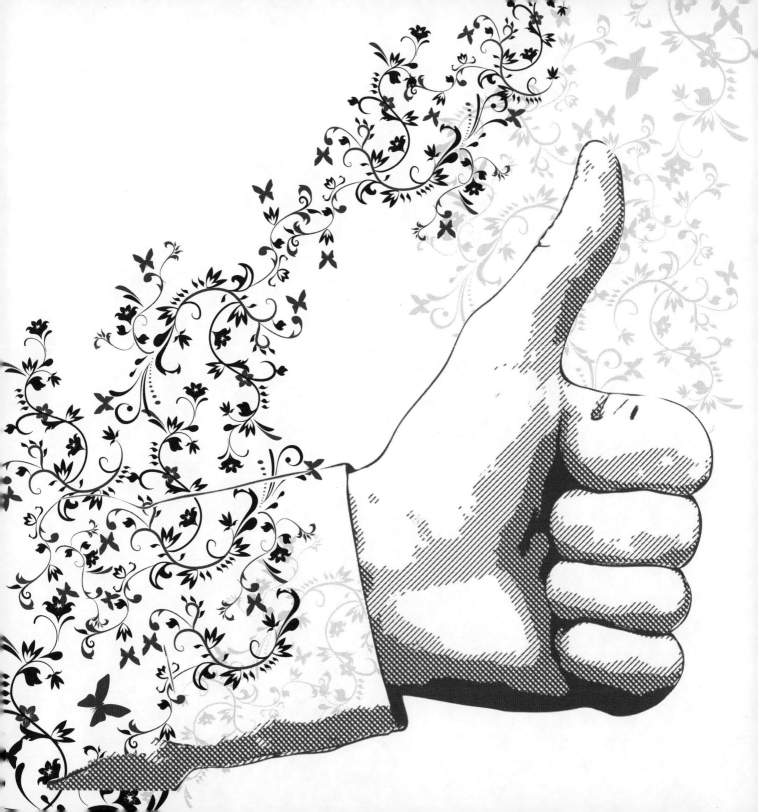

Under My Thumb

— Dr. Mary —

Definition: Frumpy

A girl or woman regarded as dull or plain, colorless and primly sedate.

Urban Definition: Frumpy

A female figure who is chunky... but not to the point that she is a "lard."

discovered that when I told my patients to go vegan, they would give me a look of horror and immediately start searching their smart phones for the name of their next doctor. I now try not to use any "v" words on the first appointment. It's like talking about your crazy relatives on the first date. Sometimes it's better to sneak up on folks a little bit.

It's Not in the Palm of Your Hand

Cutting back on meat sounds much more appealing to my patients than giving up meat completely. But with extensive research showing that red meat significantly increases the risk of chronic disease, it's clear that reducing meat consumption to zero or near zero is best. Getting there sometimes takes time. When my patients come back six months later bragging that they have reduced consumption to a half a chicken breast each night, well, that's good progress, but it's just not going to do the trick. Eating a meat portion the size of the palm of your hand keeps your portion at about 4 to 6 ounces per day, which is promoting heart disease and cancer for sure. This is an old guideline that needs revamping, right *away*. Consider reducing meat consumption through a series of different hand measurements.

Trimming back on meat consumption is easy with this little trick. When you're making dinner, make an "OK" sign with your hand, and fit your serving of meat into the little circle. That should be a little less than two ounces. By U.S. standards, that's a laughable, puny, miniscule portion of protein. By European standards, you would be considered a moderately heavy meat eater. By world standards, eating two ounces of animal protein daily is considered an incredibly indulgent and rich diet. It all depends on your perspective.

A Wake-Up Call

~ Michelle Johnston

Five years ago, I was pretty sure that I was the picture of nearly perfect health. As a widow, standing at five foot two and a half, my blood pressure and cholesterol levels were normal, and I wore a size six petite, sometimes even a four! I was hitting all the health markers despite my high-pressure, sedentary lifestyle as a college dean. I spent most days sitting on my desk chair staring at a computer, in my car, at meetings and attending conferences. I also sat at a lot of luncheons, dinners and banquets. Being Dr. Mary's patient for almost as long as she has been in practice, and listening to her discuss plant-based diets and exercise, I often thought about making a life-altering transition to a healthier lifestyle, but I never actually did anything. I didn't think I had to.

My transition, like Dr. Mary's wake-up call, actually started with the blood test result indicating that I was pre-diabetic. As a reaction to the diagnosis, I had a ridiculous question: How could I be pre-diabetic when I wore a size six petite? Similar to Dr. Mary's reaction, I was haunted with a vision of becoming an old and blind amputee. I didn't want to miss out on life, especially on future adventures with my truly neat sons, both in their 30s. They were my prime motivations as I started moving toward a plant-based diet.

Just like Dr. Mary suggested, I started with meatless Mondays to start my journey. Pretty soon other days of the week became meatless too, with dishes like multigrain pasta, pesto, sundried tomatoes, and roasted pine nuts. I can't

report that my diet is completely plant-based, but it is moving in that direction. My diet is probably a cross between traditional Mediterranean and Asian diets, with heavy doses of vegetables.

This cross-international diet is not hard for me to follow while on the job. At banquets or luncheons, without a vegetarian option, I eat the vegetables, fruit and a whole wheat or rye roll. I also do my best to skip desserts. During the eating periods before the keynote speakers, I move around between the tables to greet people. It is my "move, don't eat" theory.

I also introduced soy milk into my diet, drinking a glass enriched with vitamins and calcium every morning for an extra boost of calcium. I replaced soy milk for cow's milk in my pancakes and serve my guests soy milk for their coffee.

In one of her posts, Dr. Mary discussed the effects of white, refined flour, especially on the waist. Consequently, I now eat whole wheat and multigrain products, including bread, pasta and pancake mix. Truth be told, multigrain pancakes and pasta are much tastier than the white flour version. Occasionally, I use spaghetti squash to substitute for pasta. For an elegant and

tasty entrée, I add sundried tomatoes, canned tomatoes and fresh cherry tomatoes.

In addition to eating, I changed the way that I move, using stairs rather than elevators, standing to read the paper and do evening paperwork, walking around the offices a couple of times an hour, and exercising before and after work. My exercise regimen includes stretches with a chinning bar, weights, and ball work. I also take yoga and t'ai chi lessons. When I walk, I frequently wear a weighted vest. Plus, I have a special friend with whom I can ride my electric bicycle 10 to 15 miles a day on Saturday and Sunday. For me, all of the exercises are important, but the chinning bar is especially so because I want to be the elderly lady with a beautiful posture, not stooped shoulders and a rounded back.

I didn't start this transition to lose weight. I started it to be a healthy 68-year-old who anxiously anticipates her next physical. However, I did lose about 20 pounds and sometimes find a four petite just a little baggy. My transition to a plant-based diet is not complete, nor am I. The transition and my life are works in progress.

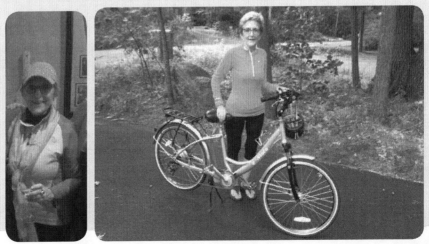

It's "OK" to Eat Less Meat

So, reassure yourself that it is "OK" to decrease meat consumption. It is "OK" to consider a plant-based diet for you and your family.

French and German nutrition researchers measure the meat consumption of their subjects on a range from vegan to heavy meat consumers. Since 1982, European researchers have studied 148,610 adults for the Cancer Prevention Study. Their research found that vegetarians are 40 percent less likely to develop cancer compared to meat eaters. They also determined that subjects with the highest meat intake had an approximately 30 percent to 40 percent higher colon cancer risk. This data adds to an already impressive body of alarming data regarding red meat consumption.

The most interesting part of the study, in my opinion, is the definition of a "heavy" meat eater, according to French and German researchers. They defined a heavy meat-consuming male as a man consuming 3 ounces of meat daily. Heavy meat consumption in women was defined as just 2 ounces of meat a day. When you begin to consider reduction in meat intake, consider the definition, and consider the source of the dietary guideline you are following.

Under Your Thumb

You can consider your meat consumption under control when you've got it under your thumb. Fit your daily meat portion under your thumb and you will be incredibly close to achieving vibrant health. According to Dr. T. Colin Campbell, getting 95 percent of your calories from plants is just as good as getting 100 percent of your calories from plants. Campbell, the author of more than 400 studies on nutrition during his tenure at Cornell University, also states that if you are eating a 2,000 calorie per day diet, you should be able to consume 100 calories per day of animal protein without significant health consequences. For me, that translates to an occasional non-vegan bakery item. It translates into not interrogating a friend about the use of chicken broth or eggs in her cooking when I'm eating at her house. For others—who don't eat any animal product for ethical as opposed to health reasons—the calories aren't really an issue. In fact, even one calorie is too much.

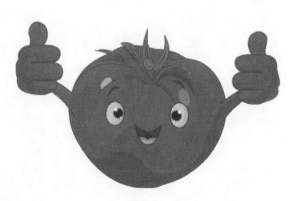

Eating 100 percent plants is still the best. Kathy Freston, author of The Lean, argues for progress, rather than perfection, in transitioning to a plant-based diet. You can get there easily by taking your favorite recipes and replacing meat with whole grains and beans, which are the concentrated calorie powerhouses of the plant community. Please don't waste a lot of time getting there, though. Remember that's it's "OK" to consider some dramatic changes to your diet. Soon, just as Mick Jagger so famously found his troublesome girl, you will have your meat consumption under your thumb.

Faux-Get the Meat

Some people find it easier to transition to a vegan diet by replacing their meaty favorites with plant products that taste pretty darn close. Remember my barbequed rib addiction? Jiminy Crickets, did I miss barbequed ribs! When I found the faux ribs in my grocer's freezer, I stared at them for a long time before I finally bought them and brought them home. They are delicious! I don't know how the company makes plant products so tasty. When I was making my transition, eating those ribs made things a little better. Nowadays, I'm a long way away from pining over a missed meat meal. Choosing faux corn dogs, veggie burgers and ribs made the transition pretty easy, especially at barbeque get-togethers where you can feel a little left out and hungry. But some of these products are processed and high in fat, and should not be considered a routine part of a healthy plant-based diet. But

by leaning on them early in your transition, you can get your meat consumption under your thumb more quickly. That translates to dramatic reductions in multiple chronic diseases, in study after study.

The Skinny on Getting Healthy

Once you become a committed vegan, chances are your extra pounds will drop off effortlessly—especially if you exercise 30 minutes every day, or nearly every day. Let's face it, you'll be skipping steaks, ice cream, cheese, butter and donuts—the stuff that not only puts rolls on your belly, but also can make you sick.

That's not just my opinion. Dr. Joan Sabaté, who heads up the Department of Nutrition at Loma Linda University in California, analyzed multiple studies and found that, on average, vegetarian men weigh an average of nearly 17 pounds less than their meat-eater counterparts. Vegetarian women weigh 7 pounds less. And vegans are even skinnier. An article in the International Journal of Obesity says that meat eaters have the highest body mass index, followed by vegetarians and then vegans.

If we part the curtain a little bit and glimpse some hard truths, we Americans eat a lot of meat and a good share of us are fat. More than one in three Americans are considered obese. Consider that the average American gets 67 percent of his or her dietary protein from animal sources, just about twice of the world-wide average of 34

percent, according to Polly Walker, the lead author in "Public Health Implications of Meat Production and Consumption" published in the March 2, 2005, issue of the *Journal of Public Health Nutrition*.

I'm going to go through a few studies that basically reflect the fact that vegetarians, on average, are sleeker. In the Swedish Mammography Cohort study, researchers asked 55,459 women whether they considered themselves omnivores, semi-vegetarians, vegans or lacto-ovo vegetarians (they eat products with milk, but not eggs or cheese with rennet or yogurt with gelatin). Here's how the overweight percentages broke down: omnivores (40 percent); semi-vegetarians and vegans (29 percent); and lacto-ovo vegetarians (25 percent).

Now, observational studies are criticized because there could be other things at work. Maybe vegetarians weigh less because those types of folks tend to eat healthier foods overall and exercise more.

So let's also take a look at the Cancer Research study in the United Kingdom, in which 22,000 folks were tracked for five years. Those in the study that started and ended as meat eaters and fish eaters put on more weight over a five-year period than the study subjects who switched over from meat eating to vegetarianism. The nice thing about this study is that you're comparing before and after outcomes with the same set of people.

The study concluded that we all put on weight as we age, but vegans and vegetarians put on the least weight of all—an average of .5 kilos (1.1 pounds) compared to the overall average of 2 kilos (4.4 pounds).

Those who were physically active during the study gained even less.

So folks eating a diet high in carbohydrates and low in protein are simply skinnier. Take that Dr. Atkins! But if you want to step up your weight loss even more, I'll talk about calories in the next chapter.

You Need to Make Up Your Mind

~ Helen Lutz

Hi, I'm Helen and 73 years young.

I had my yearly physical with Dr. Mary Clifton in 2006 and was advised that my sugar level was slightly elevated, and that I needed to watch my sugar intake (I weighed 175 lbs.). I learned about diabetes when I was in nurse's training and I had a really hard time with the diabetic diet. I did not want to be diabetic, so I decided that on this day, I would take obvious sugar out of my diet. No more soda pop, cookies, cherry pie or chocolate. Dr. Clifton was pushing a vegetarian diet, so I thought I would try to do this also. No more beef, bread, fast food. Losing weight was not my primary concern—not being diabetic was. The weight came off naturally.

My daily diet now for breakfast is a V-8 juice and oatmeal with a small amount of dried cherries with no milk. Lunch is usually a vegetable or a salad. Sometimes my husband will share a small piece of the chicken or salmon he has on his salad.

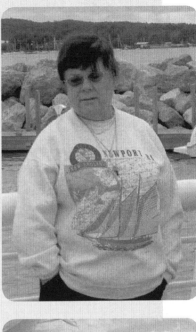

I only drink hot or cold water, no more coffee or caffeine. I take a dietary supplement powder mixed with 8 ounces of soy milk. This gives me my protein, multivitamins, mineral and digestive support. I eat small portions and never eat anything after 6 PM.

I developed arthritis in my knees, as well as a pinched nerve in my right hip, which forced me to curtail my walking outside. I started walking on a treadmill 3 hours a day and now I'm up to 4 and a half. My speed is 2.3 miles an hour, with in incline of 3.5. I have been keeping track of my miles and the calories burned since January 1, 2012. I walked 1106 miles the first six months of the year and burned up 261,264 calories. My weight now is 114 lbs.

Losing weight is in your mind; you must make up your mind completely to lose weight. Take small portions of food. When you lose weight, the only way you can keep the weight off is to eat the same way you did while losing the weight.

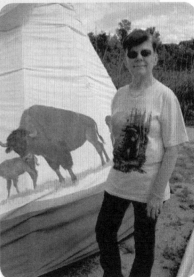

"Dr. Mary Clifton Changed My Health and My Life"
~ Paul Goodman

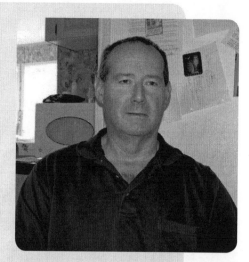

I have been diabetic since 1977. At that time, I weighed more than 325 pounds. Over time, my weight went up and down, but I could never keep it under 200 pounds. My food cravings centered on chocolate, snack foods and soda. Over time, my health problems increased and included high blood pressure and back pain. All my doctors wanted me to follow a portion-controlled, diabetic diet based on the typical American diet.

Dr. Mary Clifton changed my health and my life. At age 55, I was taking several medications, weighed more than 250 pounds and was walking with a cane. At my first appointment, she recommended that I switch to a plant-based diet with exercise. I was willing to try it since no other diet seemed to control my weight.

The first two weeks were the hardest. I seemed to crave foods like turkey, and macaroni and cheese. After that, I found it easier to stick with, and I noticed that I was losing weight. Eventually, the weight seemed to "melt" off without really trying. From the beginning, I started to walk, and increased the distance each week. Several months later, I was within my target weight and am continuing a plant-based diet. At my request, the doctor said that an occasional "treat" was ok, such

as chocolate or meat. I have found that I don't really crave those things anymore. Chocolate is easy to pass up. I only have meat when friends have me over for lunch or dinner. I always eat more vegetables than any other food and prefer it. My favorite "combo" is rice/beans/garlic.

If my memory is correct, I have been off of almost all medications for almost two years, except one pill for blood pressure.

I realized during the process that the food I had eaten all my life was a habit—we eat what our parents feed us, which is "normal" for us. Food habits are part of our culture, I think. My mom's typical dinner was "meat and potatoes." My biggest concern was getting enough protein, but with the doctor's guidance, I mixed grains with beans and legumes. I've also found that raw fruit or vegetables seemed to suppress my appetite somewhat. In retrospect, changing my diet was not difficult.

I knew that if I didn't make a change, I could die an early death and I wanted to live—actively. And now I do. I walk and bicycle and play with "toys" such as jet skis, ATVs and snowmobiles. My days of using a cane are long behind me.

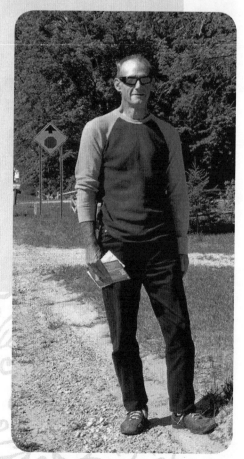

Pink Bean, Quinoa and Spinach Soup

An appetizing, mildly spiced mélange of nourishing beans, grains, and greens, this makes a stellar centerpiece for a soup-based meal, as it's done in 30 minutes or less. Quinoa is an excellent source of protein, making this practically a meal in a bowl.

Nava Atlas is an amazing vegetarian chef. She's the author of several cookbooks and a regular contributor to DrMaryMD.com's weekly recipes. She's especially good at preparing soups and stews. I hope you enjoy this recipe as much as me and my family do. *Recipe adapted from Vegan Express.*

Serves: 6 or more

1 1/2 tablespoons extra virgin olive oil
1 medium onion, finely chopped
8 baby carrots, quartered lengthwise
2 cloves garlic, minced
2 natural, salt-free vegetable bouillon cubes
2/3 cup quinoa, rinsed
One 15-to 16-ounce can pink beans, drained and rinsed
2 teaspoons good-quality curry powder
Pinch of cinnamon
Pinch of ground nutmeg
3 medium tomatoes, diced
5 to 6 ounces baby spinach leaves, well rinsed
Salt and freshly ground pepper to taste

Heat the oil in a large soup pot. Add the onion and sauté over medium-low heat until translucent. Add the carrots and garlic, and continue to sauté until all are golden, about 5 minutes.

Add 6 cups water, followed by the bouillon cubes, quinoa, beans, and spices. Bring to a rapid simmer, then cover and simmer gently for 15 to 20 minutes, or until the quinoa is tender.

Stir in the tomatoes and cook for 2 to 3 minutes, until they soften. Add the spinach and cover. Cook for just a minute or two, until it is wilted, then stir it in. Adjust the consistency with a little more water if the soup is too dense; season with salt and pepper and serve.

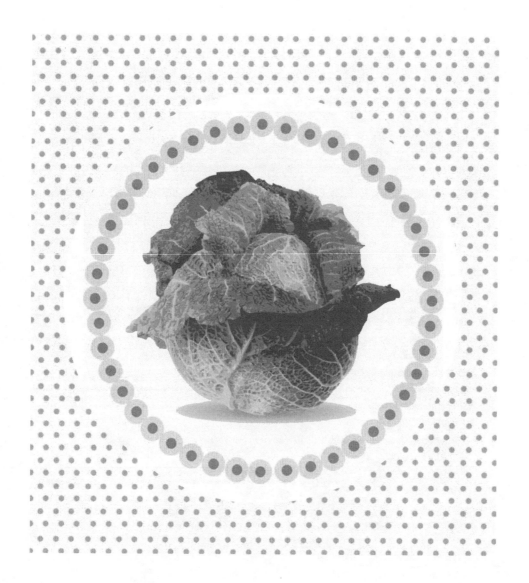

Counting Down Your Pounds

— Dr. Mary —

Streamlining your diet by consistently reducing calorie intake by 100 calories a day will result in weight loss of a pound a month. At the end of the year, that adds up to 10 pounds. If you think about it that way, very simple modifications to your diet can add up to big results.

*L*et's imagine that you like to drink coffee with cream and sugar. If you drink two or three cups per day, you are easily ingesting 100 calories of inflammation and cancer-promotion.

Switching to three cups of green tea per day results in increased serum levels of cancer-fighting antioxidants and cuts calorie consumption by a hundred calories a day, leading to a pound of weight loss a month. This calculates to a 10-pound weight loss in a year. A gal can get a nicer, trimmer silhouette in a relatively short time, without a lot of misery and deprivation.

Sugar's Not So Sweet

But there is more to the numbers than just calories. That's the contention of Gary Taubes, author of *Why We Get Fat* and *Good Calories, Bad Calories*. He argues that not all calories are created equal and points to high-fructose corn syrup and sucrose (that pretty white sugar you use to make cookies) as the culprits behind our country's widening waistlines. His argument goes like this: If you chemically break down high-fructose corn syrup (HFCS) and sucrose, you'll find that both are made up of a nearly 50/50 share of glucose and fructose. The good thing about glucose is that every cell in your body can metabolize it. Not so with fructose, which is metabolized mostly by your liver cells. Some of the fructose is converted into fat and the fat collects in your liver cells. When that happens, your liver cells won't accept insulin as easily. The medical term is these fat cells become "insulin resistant." When that happens, your body naturally amps up the insulin production to compensate. Higher insulin levels means a steady trickle of added fat to your lovely body every day, and eventually that daily trickle adds up to really significant pounds at the end of the year.

So bottom line, fructose and sucrose, bad. Glucose, fattening, true, but not as bad. There was a study at the University of California Davis that confirmed this. Researchers took 32 overweight and obese men and women and required them to drink a measured amount of energy drinks over 12 weeks—30 percent of their energy requirements with each of their three meals. One group was given fructose-sweetened energy drinks, while the other control group was given glucose-sweetened drinks. Both groups gained about the same amount of weight during the twelve weeks, but only the fructose group suffered unhealthy changes in their liver function and fat deposits. Researchers, measuring insulin and lipid levels in rigorous blood tests, found that the fructose group had become more resistant to insulin—an early sign of diabetes. Their bodies also trapped more visceral fat, the nasty kind that gets into the tissues between the heart and liver and other organs, as well as secreting hormones that mess with your metabolism and leads to hardening of the arteries and heart disease. The results were published in the December 2008 *Journal of Clinical Investigation*, if you'd like to read more. Bottom line, when you choose to cut 100 calories, cut the sweet stuff first.

Be Saucy

Another easy way to trim calories is to eliminate processed dairy products. Mexican food tastes fresher and lighter without a layer of cheese on the top. A hot baked potato is delicious with mustard or steak sauce, chives and mushrooms, instead of a dollop of sour cream and butter melting down the side. Vegetables are wonderful with a light salt and pepper garnish instead of buttery sauce. Fruit smoothies taste fantastic with some orange juice or ice cubes for liquid volume instead of milk or yogurt.

My favorite personal conversion happened at our local steakhouse, where I used to chow down on big slabs of beef prepared rare and served with lots of steak sauce. After my conversion to a vegan diet, I missed those delicious steak dinners very much. I would eat a salad and a dry baked potato and feel frustrated and deprived. One night, after ordering my potato and exhaling a big, long sigh of restriction and deprivation, I realized that I didn't love the steak. I loved the steak seasoned well with salt and pepper, covered with several mushrooms and dripping with steak sauce. I called the waitress back, and asked her to add a side of mushrooms and

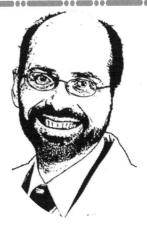

MERCURY IN CORN SYRUP?

—MICHAEL GREGER, MD

CREATOR OF WWW.NUTRITIONFACTS.ORG

The corn corporations say there's no mercury. Fact... or fiction?

Fiction: In a study that attempted to answer everything you wanted to know about high fructose corn syrup but were afraid to ask, researchers looked at 50 different brands, from soda pop, to pop tarts to yogurt.

The results? Thirty percent of these foods with high fructose corn syrup were contaminated with mercury, and it was 60 percent for the dairy foods. An average woman of childbearing age eating these products every day would consume the EPA's safe upper limit. So, we probably shouldn't let our kids become children of the corn. Of course a can of tuna may have as much mercury as an entire gallon of high fructose corn syrup, but still. Taking the mercury content into account, high-fructose corn syrup is worse than sugar, but neither is good for you. They are both just empty calories—calories, with no nutrition.

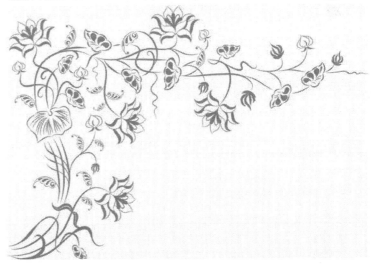

bring the steak sauce. Then I cut up my homely little plain potato, covered it with salt and pepper and chives, mushrooms and steak sauce. I ate like royalty.

Now, I go to the steakhouse craving my delicious dressed-up potato. It is so creamy and decadent in all of its layered flavors, I don't miss the steak and butter and sour cream at all. No kidding! The kids have fun teasing me about my potato addiction, and that's fine because I have a lot of fun eating it. Everybody wins.

At first, I craved my old favorite meat dishes. I soon realized that they were so delectable because of all the fuss that got put into preparation of the meat. The layering of flavors through seasoning, marinating, grilling, and saucing makes the meat very delicious. A great meal meal is defined mostly by the flavors, and not by the cut of meat. If you pop a veggie burger on the grill next to the meats and cover it in barbeque sauce, you can live it up just like the omnivores. Layering the flavorings and seasonings of vegetables and taking advantage of marinades, can make ordinary vegetables very appealing.

Wishful Thinking

I used to love the smell of meat cooking on a barbeque. The smoky, rich aroma was irresistible. I didn't know how I could ever break that craving. Then I read about movie stars who made negative associations with foods to help end their desire for the food. For example, you might now take a bite of cheese and savor the cold creaminess on your palate. You might like the sharp initial flavor that sweetens over time. Heather Locklear had a similar problem with excessive consumption of bread. I have no problem with anyone eating a lot of bread, since great whole grain bread is good for you. I have a problem with the stuff all you gorgeous gals are putting on the bread. Our country is in a low-carb craze, though, and Heather thought it made sense to cut out bread. So she thought about smog every time she had a bite of bread in her mouth. By associating something very yummy with something very yucky, she stopped having such terrible cravings for the food.

The same thought process has worked amazingly well for me and my love for barbeque. When I smell it, and I start to feel the old temptation return, I think of dirt and feces. I think of a tender little pig in a crate on a factory farm, never knowing a big gulp of fresh air or the feel of his nose rutting around in some good mud. If that seems like too much to imagine, you could do something as simple as imagining a mouthful of smog when you are eating a mouthful of meat. It's easier to avoid meat when you connect the right thoughts to consumption.

I used to make the most delicious Vietnamese pork bundles in the old days, when I ate meat. They were made with ground up pork, mounds of fresh shredded ginger and chopped garlic, chopped peanuts and lemongrass. They were absolutely delicious. A sprinkle of Vietnamese *Must-Have Table Sauce*, a combination of fish sauce with vinegar and sugar, set the flavor off perfectly. I mourned the loss of those little treasures from my diet for four years. About a year ago, I stood in my kitchen in front of my stove trying to determine what I could cook for dinner. I realized that I could substitute the pork with some pinto beans. Their creamy goodness and their coloring after cooking approximates ground pork reasonably well. I filled my house with all the delicious smells of Vietnamese cooking, bringing my children up from their electronic television and computer marathon in the basement. Ice Daughter is too young to remember the smells and arrived with a curious expression on her face, wondering what could possibly be for dinner. Number One Daughter gulped big smells of the kitchen air and proclaimed, "I miss you cooking like this!" and took over the preparation of the table sauce. She mixed rice vinegar, sugar and a little salt in place of the fish sauce together, and soon dinner was served. The healthy, transformed lettuce bundles were mouth-watering and utterly delicious. The girls enjoyed all the cancer-fighting and weight-controlling benefits that a diet rich in beans, vegetables and nuts provides.

Dr. Mary's Must-Have Table Sauce

¼ cup fresh lime juice

¼ cup fish sauce (I've substituted ½ teaspoon salt for the fish sauce, and I think it tastes better plus it keeps the recipe vegan)

¼ cup water

2 teaspoons rice or cider vinegar

1 tablespoon sugar

1 small garlic clove, minced

Optional: One bird chili (a tiny Asian chili) or 1/ cup of jalepeno, seeds removed), and minced, carrot shreds.

Mix all your ingredients in a bowl, stirring vigorously to dissolve the sugar. Top with optional chili and carrot, if you like. Keeps refrigerated for three days.

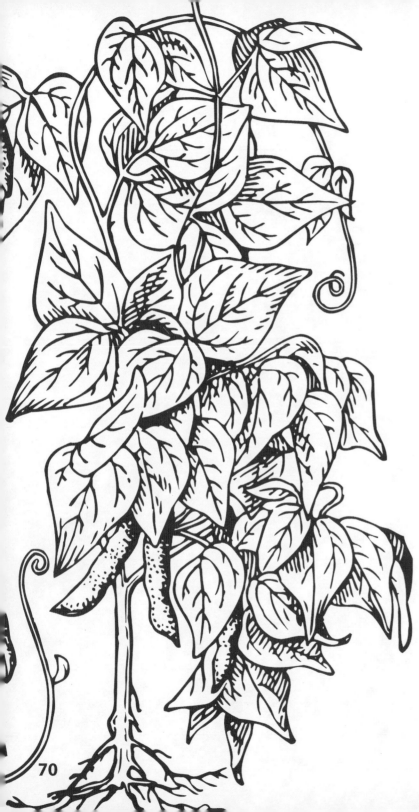

Beans To Go

Everywhere you put meat, you can put a bean. Beans have as much protein as meat, calorie for calorie. Layer flavors and seasonings on your beans, and you've made a dish to crave for! In addition, there are multiple different tasty beans to choose from when you are creating new dishes.

In Mexican food, a stout little black bean is the perfect substitute for hamburger or pulled pork. In soups, kidney beans and pinto beans seem to maintain their shape after prolonged cooking. In hummus and dips, garbanzo beans have a creamy texture after food processing or blending that resembles the unhealthy sour cream/cheese dips you are working so hard to replace in your diet. For an incredible taste, add dried cherries and chipotle! Beans have a variety of flavors and textures and colors that make rubbery dry chicken breasts look, well, boring.

Beans are great, but don't forget to spotlight all the other delicious vegetables and fruits in your diet. As you push meat and dairy off your plate, you can add bigger servings of veggies and sweet potatoes (healthier than regular potatoes). Scour the Internet for all kinds of tasty recipes for your vegetables.

Consider making a creamy potato au gratin with dairy-free milk and cheese substitutes. Touch your freshly steamed asparagus with an immersion blender and finish with a little sea salt for a delicious, refreshing spring soup. Make a veggie-rich quesadilla with a little hummus replacing the diary, to hold all the veggies in place, and enjoy the crispy goodness of toasted whole grains with fresh salsa.

Trim your plate of all that extra fat by choosing alternatives for animal products in your favorite dishes, and then you will happily notice a trimming of your waistline in a very short time. It's easy to do when you trim 100 calories at a time.

Dr. Mary's Veganized Pinto Bean Bundles

(With special thanks to the cookbook, Hot Sour Salty Sweet: A Culinary Journey Through Southeast Asia, for inspiration!)

I 12-ounce can of pinto beans

1 tablespoon tamarind pulp, dissolved in ¼ cup warm water

1 tablespoon walnut oil

½ cup chopped shallots

3 tablespoons minced garlic

2 tablespoons brown sugar

½ to 1 teaspoon salt

1 tablespoon minced ginger

2 tablespoons dry roasted peanuts, finely chopped

Rinse and drain beans thoroughly in a colander. Set aside. Whisk the tamarind and water together, then discard the pulp.

Heat your large frying pan or wok. Add oil, shallots and garlic. Stir-fry until golden. Then add the beans. Stir until heated through. Add the sugar, salt, tamarind juice, and cook until the liquids have almost evaporated, or around five minutes. Add the ginger and peanuts and cook for just 30 seconds. You may add a bit of salt or sugar if you like.

To make a bundle, put some of the yummy bean mixture into a romaine lettuce leaf. You could sprinkle with a pinch of fresh chopped scallions. Wrap the lettuce leaf around the beans and enjoy!

We usually make Must-Have Table Sauce to accompany the wraps. Each diner gets their own little bowl and spoon, since this sauce is meant to be spooned on the food bite-by-bite, according to the diner's personal preferences. I use my ramekins, positioning one at the top right of each table setting, with a few carrot shreds floating atop the Must-Have Table Sauce.

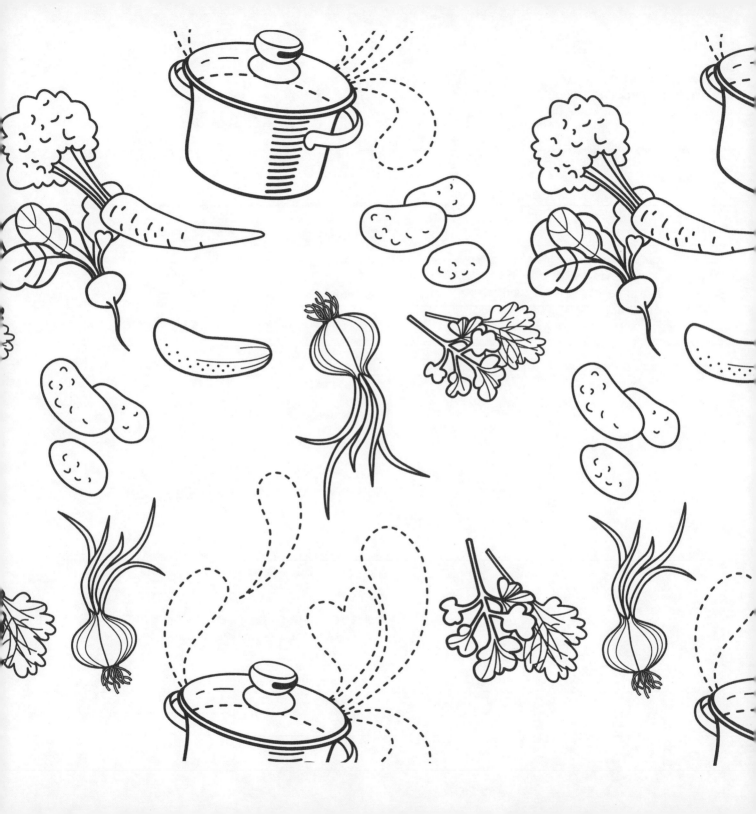

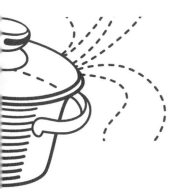

The Art of
Not Snacking
— Dr. Mary —

The possible benefits or drawbacks of regular snacking are hotly debated in the nutrition literature. Many people think that several small meals a day will help maintain a normal body weight, because they feel less hungry and may eat less food at mealtimes.

If you look at trends over the last 50 years, it would seem that these suggestions to eat more frequently, supported, interestingly, by the snack food industry, have done their job. Americans have effectively increased their number of meals and snacks each day. In the 1960s, Americans were pencil thin. On average, we ate three times daily. There were strong societal prohibitions against gluttony, and very few people thought it reasonable to eat four times a day. Many people ate just twice a day, and some even admitted to eating just once a day.

Now, the average frequency of eating is up to five times a day. This includes breakfast, lunch, dinner and a snack during the day. In addition, a little late night snack in front of the TV is thrown in there, too. There are very few people eating just three times a day, and some people are eating 7 or 8 times daily, which is essentially continuous consumption of nutrients, little bits of snacking all day long.

The idea of routine snacking doesn't seem to be working for the average American. The problem is, most of us are eating healthy at mealtimes. A bowl of oatmeal for breakfast, a big salad or veggie wrap at lunch, and some stir fry for dinner is a very balanced, healthy diet. These healthy meals are not going to support extra weight or chronic disease. The problem with snacking lies in the foods we select for snacking.

If we selected raw vegetables as a healthy snack, we would be fine. Vegetables can be eaten without consideration for caloric content, because they are so low in calories that a person would fill up way before they ate too much. There really is no definition of excess vegetable consumption, and no upper limit of vegetables that would negatively affect your health. The only vegetable exception to this rule is potatoes, since potatoes do have considerable calorie concentration and are often not eaten raw, but rather sliced and fried in the form of chips or French fries. If a snacker chose to eat just raw vegetables when snacking, no problem!

But I'm here to tell you, that's just not happening. When people reach for a snack, they go for the salty, crunchy, sweet, or/and creamy—or sometimes all four at a time. Salty and crunchy snacks are comprised of things like trail mix, roasted and salted nuts, pretzels, popcorn, chips and crackers. Sweet and creamy snacks include peanut butter, cookies, candies, ice cream, sweetened coffees and smoothies. A lot of the ingredients for the snacks, of course, arrive at the factory door healthy and whole, but by the time they leave sealed up in a snappy little box, they're stripped of their fiber and water—even their natural flavors in some cases. If that isn't bad enough, they are also plumped up with fat, sugar, salt and artificial flavorings specially designed to keep you craving for—Just. One. More. Not only does the processing make them unhealthy, it also concentrates the calories, making for smaller and smaller serving sizes.

A Spoonful a Day and the Fat Comes to Stay

Now, the snacker has to decide to exercise their willpower on a highly desirable, very tasty snack, eating only a handful of potato chips or crackers, just half of a cream cheese bar, yogurt cup, or just a small scoop of ice cream. These snacks are packed with calories, with a typical spoonful of many creamy snacks approaching 100 calories. The snack industry and various weight loss organizations—and even our own government recommendations—suggest that Americans should move more and eat less if they hope to get control of their weight. But remember that just 100 calories a day in your diet will adjust your body weight by one pound a month. Increasing your snack serving by just one spoonful or one handful doesn't seem like anything, really. In the case of snacking on vegetables, it isn't. In the case of snacking chewy/sweet or crunchy/salty, it will completely undo your diet. If you choose processed snacks just twice a day and overeat on your snacks, you could gain a few pounds each month. By the end of the year, that is a 25-pound weight gain.

Look at it the other way. If you are a typical American eating five times a day, choose to simply not snack on anything but vegetables or fruit (but avoid fruit juice, which often contains fructose without any of the great fiber of fruit). Once you lose the high-calorie snacks, you will also lose an average of 300 calories per day from your diet. That's a little over two pounds a month, 25 pounds a year, which brings a woman who is dealing with a serious spare tire around her middle to fabulousness in just one short year.

Vegans are most likely not to snack on what I basically consider crap food, mainly because a lot of the bad stuff contains eggs. When there's not much to choose from, most vegans start planning ahead and bring a little container of fruit and raw veggies (maybe a side of hummus) to work. You know it's in the fridge anytime for when you're hungry, making it easy way to bypass all the donuts and cookies that people bring from home and leave in the lunchroom, along with the soda machines and vending machines with their enticing packaging.

THE POOP ON THE NEW ANTI-FAT DRUG

There's been lots of buzz about "Alli," the new over-the-counter fat-blocking diet drug. It comes with side effects of course. Side effects with names like "anal leakage." This is from the drug company's own website promoting the drug, and they are so concerned about the resulting uncontrollable diarrhea that they advise: "It's probably a smart idea to wear dark pants, and to bring a change of clothes with you to work." They are forced to advertise the fact that the drug may cause you to crap in your pants at work. So, I guess you can choose between a good diet or a good diaper.

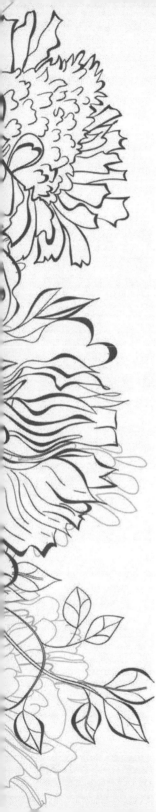

"I'm Just Not a Snacker"

For myself and patients, I prefer the "just say no" approach. Basically, you handle your urge to eat the same way you handle other urges. It's not that you don't have willpower, because I bet you are limiting your response to a virtual ton of different desirable stimuli. For example, when you are at work and you find yourself yawning at three in the afternoon, do you lay your head down on your desk and take a little nap? Probably not. You get up, walk around, maybe go outside for fresh air. And you make a note that tonight, you'll probably need to go to bed a little earlier to catch up on sleep. If you start thinking about your adorable partner in the middle of the afternoon, do you jump in your car and rush home to have sex? Probably not. You write a quick, suggestive text to your hotty before you get back to work, and look forward to some fun and intimacy later in the evening.

The same thing goes with food. If you are feeling hungry at ten in the morning or two in the afternoon, congratulations! Girls lose weight when they are hungry, not when they are stuffed. You are on the right track! You can take note of your feelings and return to work without responding to them. You can remember that food tastes the best when you get really hungry before mealtimes, and make sure that you have made adequate plans for a healthy dinner for you and everyone who is eating with you.

Real Food, Real Medicine

Now it is time to introduce my three favorite weight loss pills. Well, two of them are "pills," but one is actually a tablet.

Everyone wants a quick and easy method to jump-start her metabolism and lose weight without feeling hungry. I have just the right medications for you. Lucky for you, they are available without a prescription, and they aren't really medications in the traditional sense. They are my three secret weapons that I use all the time to keep my lower unit in good shape. They are my three favorite foods that fill me up without filling me out, so I can get plenty of nutritious food in my stomach without the agonizing guilt that comes from stuffing myself with unhealthy foods.

Cabbage

The first tablet is actually a big purple cabbage. Boy howdy, do I love cabbage— almost as much as I love finding inexpensive ways to bring colorful foods into my diet. While I found excellent sources for inexpensive orange foods in squash and sweet potatoes, greens in all the wide variety of dark green leafy veggies, I was boggled about purple foods on the cheap. I'm not on a budget, but I do like a bargain, and buying berries all year round in Northern Michigan is a pretty impressive investment. As I was pondering cheap purple produce, wandering the aisles at my local natural foods market, I ran across a purple cabbage. One filling cup of purple cabbage has just 22 calories. It has no fat and no cholesterol. One cup has 54 percent of your recommended daily allowance of Vitamin C and 85 percent of the recommended daily allowance of Vitamin K. It is also a good source of thiamin, calcium, iron, magnesium, phosphorus and potassium, and a very good source of dietary fiber, vitamin B6, folate and manganese.

The best part about cabbage is the outstanding variety of foods that can be created from such humble beginnings. Shredded cabbage forms the base for the easiest of raw foods, coleslaw. Who can forget the virtually calorie-free, but nutrient-rich and delicious, cabbage and tomato soup? Use it for your stir-fry with onions, serve over brown rice, and eat until you are ready to explode. Shred it thinly, then roast it in the oven, tossing every 8-10 minutes. After 40 minutes, put a little balsamic vinegar on the shreds. Top a little toast or healthy cracker with hummus and roasted cabbage shreds, and eat like a queen! I take this tasty little appetizer to parties and routinely have to hand out the recipe. You can also roast cabbage and potatoes with a veggie sausage for a quick weekday meal. Add it to your veggie hash in the morning. Put cabbage everywhere to increase the portion size without affecting the calorie content. If you get tired of purple cabbage, try green cabbage, or savoy cabbage, or all of the kissing cousins of cabbage, like bok choy or tatsoi. There are simply endless tasty salads and soups that are made better with the addition of a little or a lot of cabbage.

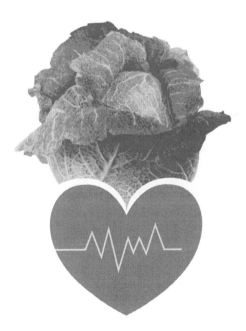

Celery

Ready for your next medicine? The tablet is actually a bunch of celery. A stalk of celery contains just ten teeny tiny calories and one whole gram of dietary fiber. Each stalk also contains 50.6 mg of omega-3 fatty acids, those wonderful, flexible fatty acids that protect against inflammation and promote healthy cellular function. While celery is not the same nutrition powerhouse as purple cabbage, it's still a good source of riboflavin, Vitamin B6, pantothenic acid, calcium, magnesium and phosphorus, and a very good source of Vitamin A, Vitamin C, Vitamin K, folate, potassium and manganese. While I don't have the diversity of recipe suggestions with celery as I do with cabbage, I love celery for its portability and ease of preparation. I particularly love it because I can eat celery until I am completely, totally stuffed and ready to lie down on the couch, and I've still probably only consumed about 100 calories.

When a girl is feeling bad after a particularly long day or when the boy doesn't call, there's nothing like a comfort food that loves you back. Stuff your face with these little stalky gems and wake up from your food coma looking even hotter on the low calories, and feeling even better on the omega-3s. Let's hope the boy that didn't call gets an eyeful of that.

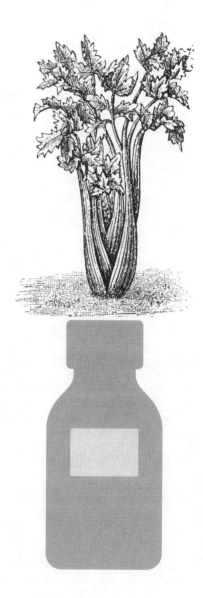

Coleslaw

Shred a half head of purple cabbage and 2 medium carrots in your food processor. Add 5 tablespoons of your favorite fat free Italian dressing. You can eat it all, or you can store it for up to four days in your refrigerator.

Cabbage Soup

2 medium sweet onions, diced (like Vidalia, walla walla etc. They have light colored skin and a slightly flattened top and bottom)

5 cloves of garlic, minced

10 oz./283 g package of mushrooms, sliced

2 tsp fresh thyme (or 1 tsp dried)

6 large stalks of celery, leaves removed and sliced

4 large carrots, peeled and sliced

1 head of green cabbage, shredded or cut with mandolin

28 oz can (or 2 16 oz cans) of fire-roasted diced tomatoes (I use Muir Glen Organics)

10 cups vegetable broth

Cook all the ingredients together in a large stockpan for one hour. Salt and pepper to taste. Store on the top shelf in your fridge for up to a week. Eat liberally without a single thought to calorie content.

Cantaloupe

As if you even need it, here's your final pill. It's the lowly cantaloupe. In fact, I think I could broaden this solitary pill into a pill packet to include honeydew and even watermelon. Melons are sweet and yet very low in sugar compared to most fruits. With 120 percent of your Vitamin A and 108 percent of your Vitamin C in a 60-calorie, one cup serving of cantaloupe, you can eat something sweet without worrying about adding pounds to your trim figure or trashing your healthy metabolism. It is also a good source of fiber, niacin, Vitamin B6 and folate, and a very good source of potassium. This summer, I've been filling the blender with watermelon and adding the juice from two limes.

As I tucked Ice Daughter into bed tonight, she requested that yummy watermelon smoothie for breakfast in the morning. I got the whole thing ready the night before and popped it in the fridge, so it was ready with just a few pulses on the blender for the Clifton girls on the go first thing in the morning. A quick puree and our breakfast was ready. I poured it into a glass of ice and garnished with some mint leaves. The simple carbohydrates in the fruit, combined with the complex carbohydrates and high fiber content, make it the perfect power breakfast for a figure skater like Ice Daughter, who needs quick energy for the first part of her workout, but also some energy that will burn more slowly and be available later in the morning too. It keeps me working smoothly all morning too.

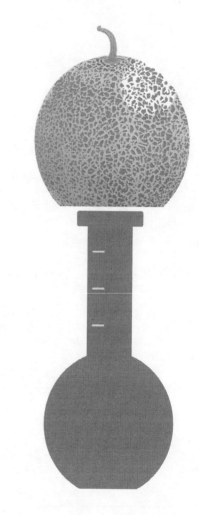

Fall in love with my favorite three fruits and vegetables, or feel free to identify a love trio of your own. Maybe you prefer fancy and unusual foods. Or exotic and expensive. Maybe your magic diet pills will include broccoli, onions and squash. That's cool. There's room for all of us in this big wide world.

Superfoods

I love to imagine the superfood and superfruits touted by the media as capable of single-handedly curing cancer, fighting chronic disease and restoring optimal health. In reality, I think the fruit or vegetable with the biggest marketing budget falls into our line of vision, whether or not it has the most benefit. If you want to think about superfoods, get together with the dieticians I hang out with at national nutrition conventions. This is a group of people who really know the antioxidant, fiber, protein and phytonutrient concentrations of various foods. Clearly, dark green leafy vegetables are the most powerful plants for fighting chronic disease and maintaining perfect health. But all fruits and vegetables, when compared to animal alternatives, are loaded with disease-preventing antioxidants and packed with filling fiber. While I love celery, cabbage and cantaloupe because of their wide availability and cheap price tag, there's a wide world of amazing and delicious fruits and vegetables right at your nearby grocery store.

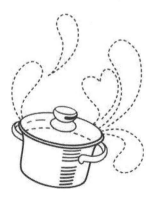

Dr. Mary's Stir-Fry

I love making this stir-fry. I make it all the time. The flavors are great together and it's quick to make when I'm hungry after work. I could eat it every day, and I sometimes do eat it for several days in a row. My parents were visiting one weekend and I took out my stovetop walk to make them my favorite dinner. Ice Daughter came stomping into the kitchen and insisted, in a very loud voice, with tiny clenched fists, that she would not eat any more stir-fry. Ever. So be careful with this one. Your family may prefer a little more variety.

In your food processor, chop ¼ head of cabbage, 3 stalks of celery, 2 medium carrots, ¼ onion, and any other vegetables or greens you have in the fridge that are starting to get a little iffy. Toss them into your wok or large frying pan with a clove of garlic and minimal oil, or better yet, a small amount of beer and rice vinegar. Cook them quickly on medium high heat for about five minutes. Add 1-2 cups cooked brown rice. Finish with a generous pour (5-6 tablespoons) of soy sauce and some crushed ginger. Add the juice of one fresh lemon if you have it. Feel free to top with a bit of hot sauce if you like. Eat a portion the size of your head.

Greens Made Easy

Wash your freshly purchased green leaves well under cold running water. Roll them up like a burrito, and then slice them very thinly. Cook them for just a minute in a hot pan with a little vegetable broth. If you are new to dark greens, you might want to add a bit of sugar, since the bitterness can overwhelm the other flavors at first. Put your freshly braised greens on a bed of brown rice or red quinoa and top with some hummus, black pepper, and the juice from half a lemon.

Make Your Own Salad Dressing

Easy! Use 2 tablespoons of your favorite jam, combined with 1/8 cup each of your favorite oil and vinegar. For example, try apricot jam with apple cider vinegar and walnut oil. Get super healthy by omitting the oil and using hummus in its place. If you prefer sweet, add a little maple syrup. You'll be surprised how little oil you need, if any, to hold the dressing together!

If It's Monday, It Must Be Broccoli

If you decide to try a plant-based diet, and you eat your vegetables like most Americans, you will find yourself very bored, very quickly. In 1996, 40 percent of Americans consumed a cake, cookie or pie every day, but only 10 percent ate a dark green leafy vegetable. Potatoes, head lettuce and tomatoes, just three vegetables, account for half of the total vegetables consumed in our country. That's no lie. If you don't look around for all the delicious variety within the plant community, you are at high risk of returning to your animal-based diet. As you experiment with new foods, try to use only one main vegetable per meal. Eat broccoli on Monday, followed by cauliflower on Tuesday, and then potatoes on Wednesday, then carrots on Thursday. By Friday, you are kinda sorta getting hungry for broccoli again. Eating different vegetables on different days keeps things fresh and interesting to you. Have you ever heard a meat-eater say that they are sick of eating chicken? I sure have. You'll get sick of these foods a lot quicker by stirring them all up together in a stir fry. Concentrating on a different fruit or vegetable each day keeps your diet fresh and fun.

The exception to this rotation is dark green leafies. If you can, gorgeous girl, eat these powerful plants every single day. If they're too expensive, grow your own. I say this casually, as though it's something that everyone can do, but I am seriously impressed with anyone who can coax food out of the ground. My neighbor across the street routinely brings five gallon buckets full of vegetables to me, leaving them outside my front door, while my own vegetable garden languishes, producing just a few new potatoes and some tomatoes that look perfect until you turn them over and see they've been attacked by some fungus or little worm. This year, I finally divided my hostas, day lilies, black-eyed susans and irises and gave them a new home where the vegetable garden used to be. I rely on my productive neighbor and our exceptional local farmers to grow fresh, enticing greens for me to nibble. Find a source you trust to develop a relationship, and get greens in your diet every day.

A Football Field of Veggies

The sheer amount of food a veg-head consumes amuses me. We eat a ton of food. It isn't unusual for me to eat a heaping plateful of salad, followed by a veggie and hummus sandwich, and to nibble on a piece of fruit for dessert. And that's just lunch. I just love to eat food.

The sheer amount of food eaten by plant-based dieters also gets in the way when my patients are trying to make lifestyle changes. The people who struggle with their weight the most will tell me with real conviction that they don't eat that much food. I believe them. The problem isn't the amount of food that they are eating, but rather the types of foods that they are choosing. If you eat a forkful of salad with a light vinaigrette, you may only consume 15 calories per forkful.

If you choose a forkful of mashed potatoes with gravy, each forkful contains 80 calories. So you can see why I eat endless forkfuls of food, while some people might be limited to just 15 to 20 bites of food a day.

It gets even more complicated than that. We each have an innate sense of how much food we should be eating, measured literally in square-footage. We know exactly how it should look as it fills up our plate. We know to the bite how much food we should consume. If we eat a little less, we've deprived ourselves. If we've eaten a bit too much, we've been gluttonous. The range of appropriate calories is surprisingly limited and narrow.

Imagine now that you've decided that some of what I'm saying here is making sense. Maybe you've gone online and looked at some undercover footage at factory farms and slaughterhouses; you've thought about the environmental consequences of your diet, and you are willing to take a leap toward better health. You are amazing. You're a rock star. You better start saving some money, girl, because you are going to need to buy some smaller clothes soon. Get ready for the best part. When you convert to a plant-based diet, you are going to have to eat a ton of food. A ton. In some cases, you may eat two or three times the square-footage of food that you eat right now.

At first, this is not a problem. You're inspired, you're excited, you're trying something new. The foods are interesting, and the weight loss is a pleasant surprise. The square-footage problem doesn't usually hit with a force

significant enough to derail your nutrition train until week six. Even though you are feeling better and losing weight, you start to feel as though you are gorging yourself. The old square-footage starts to exert itself, and soon you are practicing portion control. When you control portions on a plant-based diet, you start to get very hungry between meals. Suddenly, the diet quits working because you are hungry all the time and snacking on junk food, vegan or not, is limiting your ability to lose weight.

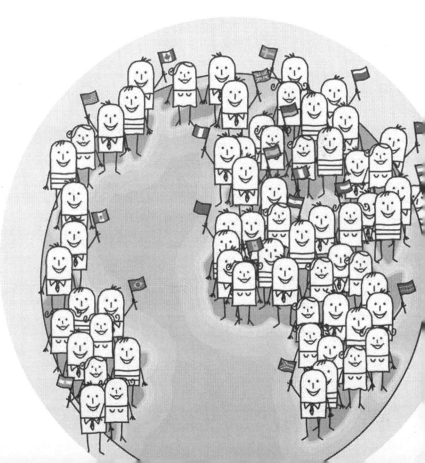

Watch out for the square-footage problem again around six months into the diet. At that point, you may have lost some serious poundage. So much so that you may need to consider some increased activity or a small calorie restriction to maintain your continued weight loss. Lots of people naturally begin to move faster and a lot more with so much less weight to carry. It becomes a pleasure to walk, run, climb stairs and chase after kids. Your metabolism revs up and the weight loss continues its nice, downward slide. But for others, the reduction in 10 or 20 pounds means a reduction in calorie burn. Your body burns fewer calories as you pursue your ordinary daily activities because it simply doesn't have to work as hard as when it was carrying 20 pounds of lard around. This slows the intensity of weight loss, and suddenly your diet program falls under tighter scrutiny. You may decide that this diet doesn't work for you, or that it is time to reconsider a low-carb option.

What Your Doctor Can Do

If you start to come undone during the sixth month of a plant-based diet, go back and meet with the professional who is assisting you in your lifestyle transformation. With most modifications, things are easy to stick with for the first four to six months. But as time passes and things become familiar, we can start to figure out a way to limit the effectiveness of the behavior we've changed. You may realize that a strict vegan diet can include potato chips, veggie chips or ice cream made from soy or coconut milks. You may find yourself plowing through a bunch of unhealthy vegan junk food and then feeling despondent when you try to slip on your skinny jeans. The best way to avoid the six-month, square-footage-trap? Distract yourself with seasonal foods.

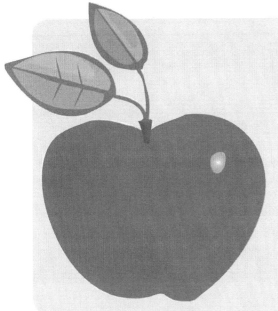

AN APPLE A DAY MEANS AN APPLE AWAY (FROM YOUR WAISTLINE)

Simply eating a great deal of vegetables, whether you're a vegetarian or not, seems to prevent an expanding waistline. When American Cancer Society researchers tracked nearly 80,000 healthy adults for 10 years, they found that men and women who ate 19 or more servings of vegetables per week did not "succumb to abdominal obesity." That is, they didn't develop spare tires. That compares to those who ate meat more than seven times a week and developed apple-shaped physiques.

The study, published in the May 1997 issue of the American Journal of Public Health, emphasized the hazards of piling on fat around the waist and developing what's known as an "apple" shape. It's more than just a cosmetic issue. An apple shape is linked to heart disease, diabetes and certain cancers.

Eat with the Seasons

Every diet gets old and boring after a few months. Last summer, Ice Daughter decided she wanted to become a fruititarian after a reading an article about ultra-marathoner Scott Jurek, who eats only fruit for weeks at a time. He reports that he smells like a citrus grove. In this particular article, he commented that if you took an orange and put it in the food processor, and he had a bowel movement in a bowl, you would not be able to tell the two apart. That comment was hilarious to my preteen, and a fruititarian was born. For a few weeks. Then, she became a fruit-and-nutitarian. Eventually, the diet collapsed and we returned to our ordinary plant-based diet.

I'm sure similar experiences could be shared in your own diet history. Our own Mother Earth knew we'd be bored with the same foods after a few short months, so she goes ahead and changes everything up every so often. If you are worried that you will be bored with a diet that limits your foods, consider eating with the seasons. You'll get plants when they are optimally fresh and delicious, and you will enjoy natural variation to your diet, the way nature intended.

How does eating seasonally look? I'm not sure why, but it looks very orange in the fall. There's a ton of squash, sweet potatoes and other root vegetables available in the fall to keep a gal feeling full and fabulous, and provide plenty of concentrated calories to get her through even the biggest jobs.

In the cold weather, our local Northern Michigan farmers keep us fed with stored roots, grains, beans and some fresh hardy greens grown in hoop houses nearly all winter long. Apples are the best winter fruit. Here at our seasonal house, though, we do indulge in a few pineapples or mangos in the middle of the winter, but these are a rare treat made particularly special by the short seasonal availability. Even though these fruits are available all year around, I don't purchase them when I have fresh, local fruit available in the summer. Pomegranates also make a short appearance in the late fall, and their red seeds are a real treat on a salad or eaten by the handful. In the late winter, the citrus returns, reminding us that we won't be in the deep freeze forever.

Once spring arrives, it's easy to find plenty of tender greens for salads. The greens and a few roots and shoots make a naturally light and refreshing diet easy to follow in the spring, when your body needs a little spring-cleaning anyway.

Summer is a wonderful bounty of delicious fruits and vegetables, with a wide array of fresh berries and fruits and vegetables. We need the extra calories too, with the addition of yard work and other outdoor activities like running and swimming and boating. The wide availability of fruit in the summer is nature's way of providing us with a healthy extra indulgence of calories to get through

our busy summer lives. Ice Daughter and I find ourselves on our bicycles riding up and down the waterfront way past our bedtimes, enjoying the long summer days and trying to figure out a way to squeeze in every last minute of sunshine out of every sweaty day.

Eating seasonally makes it a lot easier to eat healthfully. Foods naturally shift into alternate selections with the changing seasons, and healthy foods are always cheapest when they are in season. If nothing seems to be coming into season and you are still getting bored, fall back on your personal love trio for a while, and then return to the seasonal diet when you are ready.

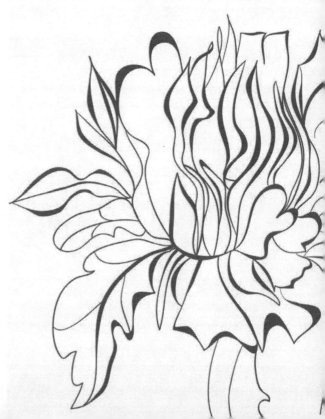

Squash Bliss

Place a whole butternut squash on a cookie sheet in the oven and bake at 375 degrees for 80 minutes. Using a paring knife and a fork, open the squash and scoop into a bowl, tossing the seeds and outer skin. Add a little date sugar (easily found in bulk online), Earth Balance Butter, and salt and pepper to taste. This is a perfectly delicious fall dinner.

Squash Soup

Using your potato peeler, peel your favorite squash. Remove any hard ends by cutting them away. Cut the squash in half, and then cut the meat of the squash into cubes a few inches wide. Place in a big soup pan with 2 apples (peeled, seeded and cut into medium-sized pieces) and one Spanish onion (peeled and cut). If you want to get crazy, put a cup of orange or apple juice in there too. Fill with 6 cups water or vegetable broth. Simmer for an hour and then blend with a heat-tolerant immersion blender.

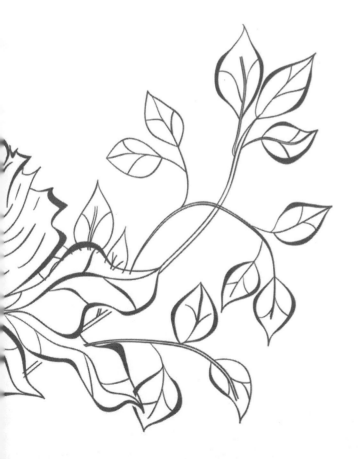

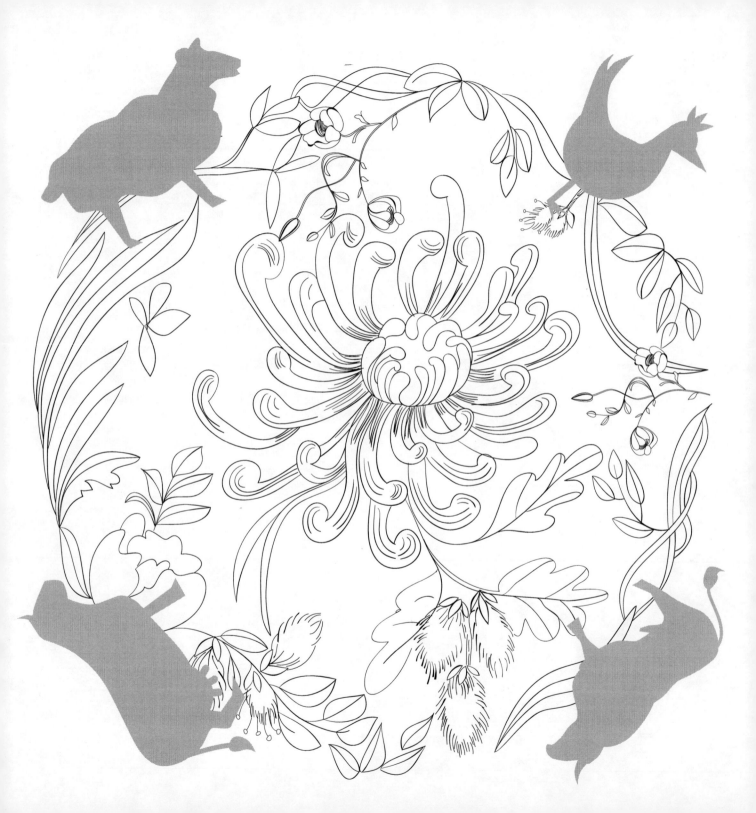

Where Do You Get Your Protein?

— Dr. Mary —

The most common question that a plant-based dieter hears from omnivores is: "Where do you get your protein?" Sometimes, after a long day of thinking and creating, I'm disinclined to visit with doubters over vegetarian sources of protein. I'll sometimes smile ironically and ask the questioner "Where do you get your fiber?" That stops the conversation about plants versus animals and allows me to enjoy myself and ignore my diet for a while.

Ignoring the question, or coming up with a snappy answer, avoids answering the underlying question, which is really the crux of the problem of adopting a vegan diet. People do have concerns about the complete nutrition in a diet that omits meat, because I think most people worry that removal of meat from the diet results in just eating salads and bread. And protein is vitally important as the building block of the body. Salads are delicious, but not particularly filling. Bread made with processed grains have the reputation for its unhealthy carbs. The trick to making successful changes that last is in the identification of concentrated calorie sources.

The question about protein is really a question about healthy concentrated sources of calories. Increasing the size of the salad and potato doesn't leave me with enough calories to get to my next meal without feeling quite hungry. The empty spot needs to get filled with whole grains like quinoa (pronounced keen-wah), brown rice, or great bread, like what we buy at our local bakery. Beans also provide concentrated calories, amazing non-inflammatory healthy protein, and a side dish of fiber, all in one little convenient package. Just a cup of bean soup provides for all the protein you need for a whole day. Fill that empty space with whole grains and beans instead of a slab of animal protein, and you will be rocking a healthy, strong body free of chronic disease in no time.

Plenty of great, anti-inflammatory protein is hiding in healthy whole foods. Spinach is 51 percent protein, mushrooms 35 percent, beans, 26 percent. Even potatoes are 11 percent protein. You may need less protein than you think. According to the World Health Organization (WHO), a 150-pound male requires only 22.5 grams of calories originating from protein. WHO also recommends that pregnant women get only 6 percent of their calories from protein. The U.S. Food and Nutrition Board recommends a daily allowance of only 6 percent after accounting for a small safety margin. Most Americans, however, are consuming protein in excess of 20 percent of their total calories, and 85 percent of those proteins are coming from animals.

Don't worry about balancing your proteins, either. Earlier research suggested that vegetarians should eat whole grains and beans at every meal, so that they can get a full complement of essential amino acids to make complete proteins. But your body is smarter than that. More recent research shows that your body is quite capable of storing amino acids for later use, when other essential amino acids become available and your body has all the necessary building blocks to create the perfect proteins for your most complex cellular processes. Instead of thinking of different foods as deficient in particular amino acids, we should consider some foods as relatively less abundant in certain amino acids. Just make sure a variety of whole grains and some beans are getting on your plate regularly. If you still worry over your protein, despite all the best data and plenty of self-education using the nutritional websites, just track your grams and take it easy. Soon you'll get a sense of what you need.

EDAMAME

Edamame are green soybeans picked before maturity, and one of my personal favorites. At 22 grams of protein per serving, they are packed with protein and super easy to prepare. Just boil them up in salt water for about six minutes, drain, add a little more sea salt and enjoy.

ABSOLUTELY SUPPLEMENT WITH VITAMIN B12—

EVEN IF YOU'RE NOT A VEGAN

I generally view vitamin supplements negatively, and I reserve recommendations for vitamin supplementation only in very limited circumstances that are not covered in the scope of this book. However, in the setting of a healthy vegan diet, the one nutrient that you may not find in abundance is Vitamin B12. Go to your local health food store and have an educational discussion with the vitamin lady. Those gals know their stuff. Choose a B12 supplement you trust and take the doggone thing all the time. I forget mine, sometimes for weeks, but I was re-energized to be more compliant after learning about the high frequency of deficiency or borderline deficiency in vegans tested in Britain. The study was reviewed on Dr. Michael Greger's website, www. nutritioninfo.org.

Vitamin B12 is made in the gut by commensal bacteria, but the quantity and continuity of this source is unreliable. It is also made by bacteria normally present in the soil. If we were still hunter-gatherers, cruising through the woods all day dining on leaves and roots, we would be getting plenty of B12 from the bacteria in the soil found on the foods you'd be eating all day long. In these modern times, we are fortunately able to scrupulously clean our vegetables and get every tiny morsel of soil washed cleanly off all of our dark green leafy good stuff. There goes the grit between your teeth, but there goes all that precious B12, too. If you quit eating even a tiny morsel of meat and became a pure vegan this moment, it would take you three years to burn through all the Vitamin B12 you have stored in your liver. The consequences of B12 deficiency include neurologic deficits, such as memory loss, dementia, numbness and tingling.

Even if you're not a vegan or vegetarian, new studies suggest the importance of taking B12 supplements owing the fact that animal products can't be relied on as reliable sources. Less than 4 percent of the B12 in scrambled eggs is absorbed, for example.

Go Get Your Protein

The idea of "protein complementarity", a concept that vegetarians must eat different proteins at a single meal in order to get quality protein, was espoused in the bestseller *Diet for a Small Planet*, way back in the 1970s, when I was still sucking my thumb. It's time to take another look at the data and banish this outdated concept.

Frances Moore Lappe' included countless charts and tables that left vegetarians struggling to understand the balance of tryptophan, methionine, lysine and other amino acids in their diets.

Basically, meat contains all the essential amino acids for protein production, but plant foods were considered deficient in one or another amino acid. Vegetarians had to balance plant foods strong in one amino acid with another plant food that was weak. The complexity of this balancing act led plenty of vegetarians to give up the effort out of fear of missing something, a concern that still lingers today. People still think that meat contains some missing ingredient that is simply not available in a healthy plant-based diet.

It's true that plant foods have more of some required amino acid than others. But virtually ALL plant foods have ALL of the essential amino acids present in more than adequate quantities to meet the needs of normal adults. Rice, for example, is relatively low in isoleucine and lysine. But rice protein provides 265% of the adult male requirement for lysine, and 266% of the required leucine. It provides 400% of the other required amino acids. Somewhere along the way, relative deficiencies got translated into deficiencies, where abundance exists.

Here's a few sample plant foods with their "limiting amino acids" listed in the percent of RDA for a normal adult male. The limiting amino acid is the amino acid contained in the lowest quantity in the food.

Limiting Amino Acid Content of Selected Foods

Corn:	Lysine 484%	Percent Calories as Protein: 15%
Wheat:	Lysine 178%	Percent Calories as Protein: 17%
Potato:	Isoleucine 241%	Percent Calories as Protein: 11%
Carrot:	Tryptophan 194%	Percent Calories as Protein: 10%

The update on complementary protein: Forget it. Eat a wide variety of foods because it's good to get a variety of vitamins and minerals, not because of protein.

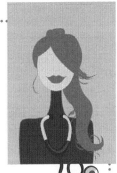

What Your Doctor Can Do
—Dr. Clinton

Testing for Vitamin B12 deficiency is readily available through your doctor. Some people become Vitamin B12 deficient despite obtaining adequate concentrations of B12 in their diet because they lack the intrinsic factor (IF), which binds with B12 in the stomach and transports it across the small intestine. Most labs will automatically check for IF when a diagnosis of B12 deficiency is made. If you are lacking it, you can take all the B12 orally you want, but you won't be able to absorb the vitamin and will still struggle with your deficiency. IF-deficient people need to obtain B12 by monthly injection or by the nifty nasal spray delivery device, which is a little more costly, but very convenient. So when you go to your next annual exam—thinner and stronger and sexier—and your doctor asks what is new, tell her about your diet. After she freaks out about your protein and calcium and scares you about eating too many carbs, politely ask her to add a B12 onto your annual labs. Tracking your vitamin B12 level may be one of the most important health interventions that a hot vegan gal can do for herself.

There is wide variability in the suggested dose of B12 necessary for supplementation by a strict vegan. I have a 1,000 mcg supplement that I take at least every other day. There are several cases of shared absorption sites for different nutrients, so I don't like to saturate all my B12 absorption sites with the vitamin everyday out of concern that the absorption sites will be rendered unable to absorb other important nutrients.

LENITLS

Lentils make a yummy soup and are also high in protein at around 17 grams per cup. Following close behind are red kidney, black, navy, haricot beans, black-eyed, garbanzo, fava, and lima beans all between 14 to 16 grams per cup.

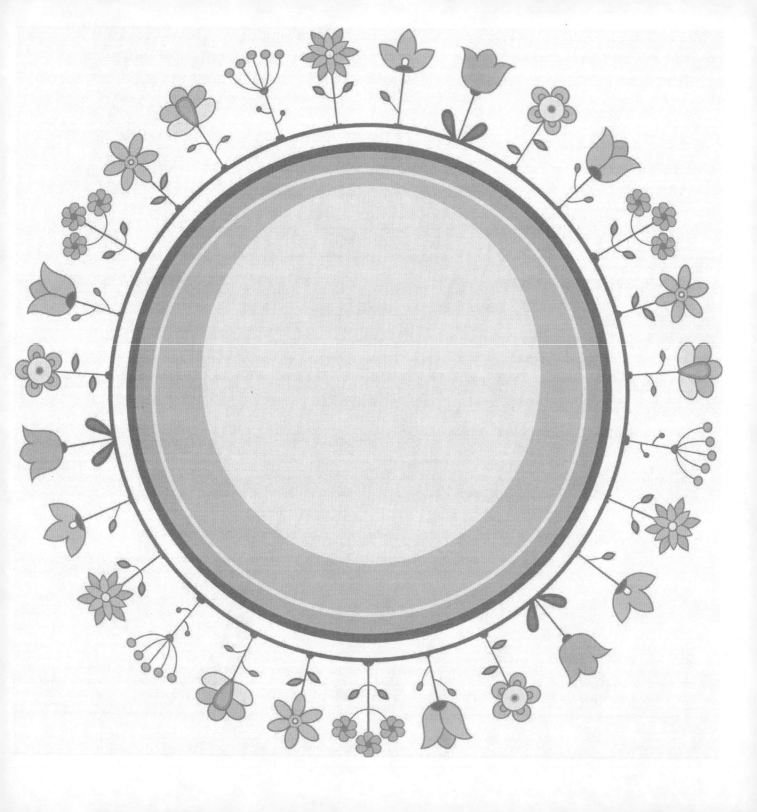

Living It Up
Dr. Mary

Right after I first started eating differently, I was invited to a lovely birthday party for a good friend. It was quite a party! Their home has a gorgeous view of Lake Michigan, and even in the winter, the icy water and snow-laden trees are magical. This was going to be quite a night. I popped into the kitchen and notified the caterers that I was going to skip the meat portion for the dinner tonight, and asked them to just bring my plate with the veggie and potato. Then I got a great glass of wine and settled into easy conversation with close friends.

We were seated at our tables and dinner was finally served. Everyone's plates were filled with slices of pork loin aside the vegetable and potato, and I waited anxiously for my good food. When my plate arrived, it had pork loin on it, too.

I immediately pointed out to the caterer that I was the gal who came to the kitchen and requested a meatless dinner. I didn't want the meat that was served to me, but I also didn't want some other gal at the party to get my meatless portion and wonder what the heck was going on. The caterer waived his hand dismissively and said, "Just eat around it." I decided that I would just eat around it and picked up my fork, but then the waiter came and whisked my plate away.

Suddenly, everyone's attention turned to me, both at my table and at neighboring tables. I had gone from being an ordinary partygoer to a pain in the butt. Everyone else's food cooled as they waited politely for my plate to return, despite my insistence that they proceed with dinner. It was moments before I was served a meatless portion, but to a social girl like me, it felt like hours as I waited for my plate. I was conspicuous, I was separating myself from my tribe, I was not accepting food that was offered to me at a celebration. Without hesitation, the questions started to come from the other partygoers about my protein. I was ill-prepared so early in my own conversion to defend my meatless decision, and now that I was being singled out, I felt more like going home and eating a container of coconut milk ice cream in front of the TV than sitting uncomfortably through dinner.

When my meal finally arrived, it arrived with the veggie and potato, and a big empty spot. Wow. I realized right then, surrounded by my friends, that this was how everyone sees my diet. I eat all the side dishes, but what goes in the big empty spot where the meat used to be? What sticks to your ribs in a plant-based diet, so you don't find yourself feeling hungry an hour after a meal? What is the concentrated source of healthy calories that leaves you satiated instead of deprived? What fills the empty spot you just created in your diet?

At the birthday party, I recovered my confidence and changed the subject by telling a ridiculous story about one of the kids, which is universally appreciated. One of my dear old friends saved the day by telling a tale of debauchery. As the birthday bo y was blowing out the candles and making a wish, I thought of a few wishes of my own. I wished I were just going with the flow, instead of sticking out like a sore thumb. I wished mostly everyone was vegan, instead of mostly everyone being omnivorous. I wished I was just like everyone else.

Become a Subscriber

Sometimes, when my interest in maintaining a healthy lifestyle starts to flounder and lose energy, I have to call on some outside help to keep me interested. I always have the latest copy of *Veg News* magazine to spark my interest. I subscribe to great websites like PCRM.org and nutritionfacts.org, so that information about healthy diets and new recipes routinely populate my emails. And, I created my own blog to help my patients get great information about diet and nutrition at their fingertips. Did you know that soda manufacturers work to get their products in front of your face at least two dozen times per day, so that you feel inclined to drink a pop? I just want to get vegan/vegetarian into my patient's minds three times a week, to keep re-igniting their interest.

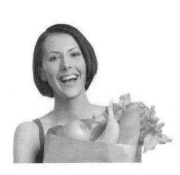

Strategies For Healthy Lifestyles

Dr. Mary
drmarymd.com

Important information for new patients

Follow Dr. Mary

Faux Flavor Flimflam

Ice Daughter and I ran across this 60 Minutes feature on flavorings, and she immediately clicked StumbleUpon to share it with the millions who find interesting content there. "The flavoring industry is the enabler of the processed food industry." True that. It's a lot easier to overeat on foods when they've been artificially salted and flavored to a higher level of desirability.

Don't Miss Anything!

Advice for Treating High Cholesterol and Obesity

A few short months ago at my hospital, I admitted a patient that was plagued with chronic nausea and headaches. I thought she had a component of lactose intolerance, and asked dietary to see her to educate her on a lactose-free diet. The dietician saw my patient. She told her that milk was a great source of calcium and protein and gave her advice on how to get even more milk in her diet. She encouraged her to never quit drinking milk, or she may be protein deficient. My patient remains sick to this day, and even more firmly entrenched in the notion that a cow's mammary secretions are a suitable food for a human woman in her seventies.

Number One forwarded me a copy of the Epocrates DocAlert on Vegetarian Diets: Five Things to Know From the Academy of Nutrition and Dietetics Research. Epocrates is a source of information for doctors that provides concise answers to specific questions. In this edition, the reviewers cover recommendations for vegetarians and dietary counseling obtained from the Academy of Nutrition and Dietetics. Here's a few of the salient points from the article:

- Vegetarians and vegans should supplement with B12. This is old news for vegetarians. B12 is manufactured by the bacteria found in food. Since vegetarians and vegans wash their produce, they wash away all the soil and healthy bacteria that are creating their B12. That's why supplementation is necessary. Meat eaters don't need to worry about their B12, because the slaughter process ensures that the meat will have lots of bacteria from poop left on it to produce plenty of B12. Even though there is plenty of controversy on where to get B12 and exactly how much you should supplement with, you should absolutely supplement with B12. Studies show that anywhere from 21% to 68% of vegans are B12 deficients. Which is cool, because when I was little and my grandma told me that I would eat a bucket of dirt over my lifetime, I almost barfed. If my diet makes me a little B12 deficient because I'm not eating dirt and poop, that's just fine with me.
- This B12 recommendation goes double for the pregnant gals.

Join the Party

This year, I went to five vegetarian festivals, all of which are incredibly energizing. Listening to amazing speakers and authors on the healthy benefits of plant-based diets and animal rights renews my energy in working on this very important issue, for my benefit and the benefit of my patients.

This year, I attended Vegetarian Summerfest (vegetariansummerfest.org) in Pennsylvania for the first time. At this event, 1,200 people converged to celebrate healthy, compassionate and ecological living. This was an event that energized this girl for a lifetime of healthy eating. The main selection area in the cafeteria was vegan. In smaller areas, there was a vegan/gluten-free/oil-free station and a raw vegan station. Ordinary eaters were encouraged not to eat from the raw vegan or oil-free stations unless they were following those diets, because choosing from these smaller areas was making it hard for the raw/oil-free folks to find enough food. Everyone was happy to comply. In addition, there were two huge salad and fruit bars at every meal. I ate watermelon three times a day for five days, which can be translated to say that I was in heaven on earth.

The North American Vegetarian Society organizes the conference, bringing together more than 65 speakers from across the country on topics regarding nutrition and health, environment and animal welfare. Attendees went to large group sessions in the morning and evening, followed by breakout sessions throughout the day. I ran, did yoga and danced Zumba with amazing chefs, boogied with authors and animal rights activists to the mixes of a vegan DJ at night, and ate vegan ice cream with national thought leaders in the nutrition community. Attending an event like this one reminded me of all the reasons that I find myself following an animal-free diet. I was so disappointed to be packing my bags on the fifth and final day of the conference, thinking about the hassles of returning home to so many unhealthy choices and so little understanding and acceptance in the general community.

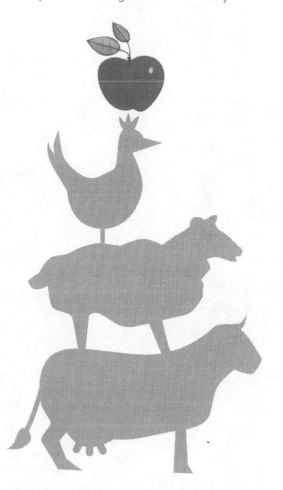

Reach Out

When you find yourself struggling in this lifestyle, reach out to other members of your vegan community. You don't need to travel to Pennsylvania to get inspired when the Internet brings all the thought leaders to your living room! When you tire of the impersonal connection you're making with the online community, check out your own community for vegetarian/vegan meet-ups and potlucks. Identify a few good people and make some new close friends, so that you can go to dinner together and support each other. Eventually, your diet will seem like the right thing to do and you'll find your way in this new, uncharted territory. Until then, lean on all these resources to help you get there from here.

So don't measure out a salad portion. Remind yourself about the square-footage trick that your brain is playing on you. Remember the lower calorie content of these healthy foods, and load up your plate so you are not ravenously hungry between meals.

We've prepared a collection of dietary comparisons in the next chapter to help you feel confident about your healthy, plant-based selections. You should feel confident, using these resources, that your nutritional needs will be met and generally exceeded with plants instead of animals. People just want to know what you are putting in your empty spot.

TONS OF FOOD

Remember the discussion on square-footage of food? Summerfest was filled with healthy people. Out of 1200 participants, I think there were perhaps six obese people. There were perhaps 20 people who had a little sticky-outy tummy or some excessively curvy hips. Everyone else was my size, or smaller. But when mealtimes came, did these people know how to put the groceries away. Everyone balanced two plates on their lunch tray, often balancing a third plate with a delectable vegan dessert on the top edge, overlapping the lips of the first two plates. Tons of food, tons and tons of food were eaten by these incredibly lean people. I can tell you that the Zumba and running and yoga classes were not that well attended. These people maintained their gorgeous figures on plants, but not by watching the portion sizes. They ate phenomenally huge portions of plants, making me giggle sometimes. I wondered how many of these converts had the same trouble with square-footage that I suffered with when I was changing my diet.

"Coming out" to Your Friends

After five years on my diet, I am still nervous about making an unhealthy selection when I'm eating out. Traverse City is now home to several small restaurants that have excellent vegan/vegetarian choices, and many restaurants will prepare a Dr. Mary Special upon request. I've only had a few chefs stomp their feet and refuse to provide me with a modified selection upon request. If I'm not at the right type of restaurant, I have to ask the waitress to write a little novel that details the modifications that I would like to my menu item. The easiest way to eat out is to choose restaurants that have great selections already on the menu. That makes it much easier to make a sane choice, without having to make your poor waitress go insane.

If you are feeling particularly uncertain about an upcoming dinner out of the house, you can always ask the restaurant to fax you a copy of the menu or review the menu online. Then, you can make your selection before you leave your house. That makes it a lot easier to avoid unnecessary temptation after your brain has been hijacked with a little drink before dinner and a couple pieces of warm, white bread.

My favorite thing about dining out is visiting with my friends and family. My second fave thing is the wonderful selection of fun wines and cocktails. I don't keep any alcohol in the house, excepting some wine for special occasions, so having a lot of different fun drinks available enhances the evening for me. I make a special deal with myself: if I make a healthy vegan selection for my dinner and I skip the bread until my salad comes, then I treat myself to a cocktail with dinner. When I first started this diet, this rule helped keep me on track while eating out. Now, it's become my lifestyle. As a special added bonus, I don't wake up feeling bloated and ashamed of all the calories I consumed while I was out with my friends. I don't feel the need to put in a huge workout at the gym the following morning, to try to avoid the bulges that come with overindulgence.

Be the Expert

As an alternative to keeping a low vegan profile, you could do research on vegan diets and arthritis, and labeling yourself the nutrition expert in your community! Being a speaker on the health benefits and ease of adoption of a vegan lifestyle makes everyone interested in what you eat, and particularly interested if you stray from your diet at all. If I wanted to eat a mess of barbequed ribs, I think I would have to go to China. Making yourself a prominent person within this movement leaves little room for error in your own diet, publicly or privately. The scrutiny of my diet has only intensified over the years. If you want to be held accountable by your community, put yourself out there as a healthy eater and let the community pressure you in that direction.

Hello!

When my daughters are about to eat in excess, I tell them, "Go ahead and eat it. No one will know, except you, and everyone who looks at you." When you work to modify your diet, and you start to feel better and look better too, everyone will want to know what you are doing and what you are eating. Everyone will suddenly become your personal nutrition expert, giving loads of free, unwanted advice. People love to talk about their health. They love to talk about their options to improve their health. They'll ask a lot of probing questions. They'll ask you about your protein. Be ready with a few short sound bites on concentrated calories and sources of protein in a vegan diet, then tell a story about one of your own goofy kids. Health is interesting, but it's not nearly as interesting as the sweet little people that are sharing your home with you.

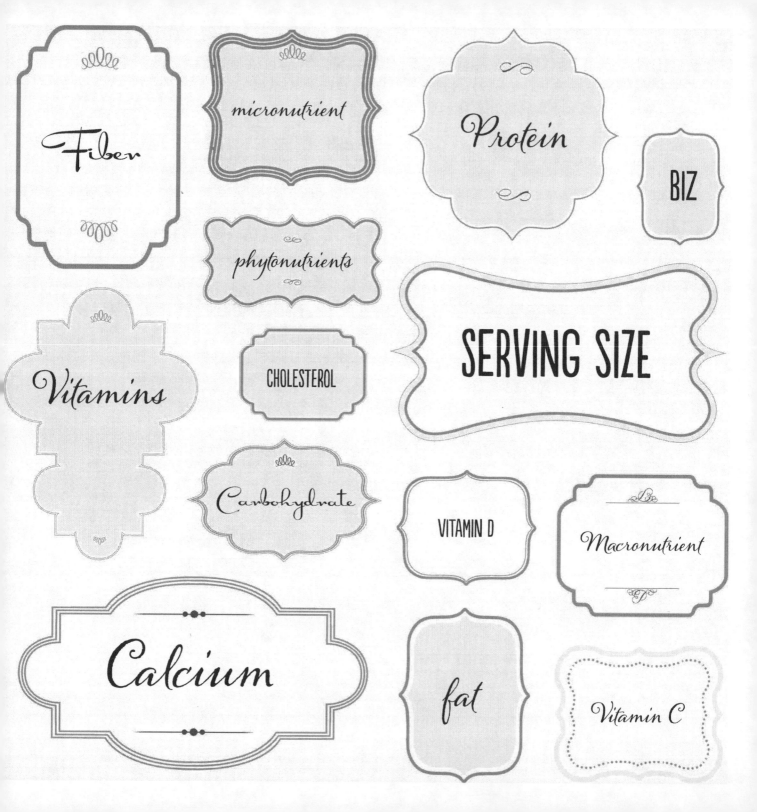

Fiber

micronutrient

Protein

BIZ

phytonutrients

Vitamins

CHOLESTEROL

SERVING SIZE

Carbohydrate

VITAMIN D

Macronutrient

Calcium

fat

Vitamin C

Read the Labels

How do meat and comparable vegetarian dishes stack up against each other? To find out, we decided to make the calorie content about equal and compare the nutrients. A sort of apples to apples approach. Plus it allows you to see how a serving size compares for the same amount of calories. For example, you can eat about 50 percent more of vegetarian chili for the same amount of calories as the meat/bean version of chili. And you get so much more of a nutritional punch!

That's why—when you lose the meat—it's so much easier to lose weight.

The nutritional labels in this chapter were compiled by MenuTrinfo™, which provides detailed nutritional information upon request for menu recipes from any restaurant. In addition to providing comprehensive nutritional analysis, MenuTrinfo™ has developed a reverse ingredient look-up and a state-of-the-art allergen identification platform to assist restaurants in developing dishes for special-needs diners. To learn more, visit MenuTrinfo™ at www.menutrinfo.com.

Burgers Comparison

Classic Cheeseburger

Nutrition Facts

Serving size 6.3 oz

Amount per serving

Calories 340

Calories from fat 170

	% Daily Value *
Total fat 19 g	30%
Saturated fat 8 g	40%
Trans fat 1.0 g	
Cholesterol 85 mg	29%
Sodium 670 mg	28%
Total carbohydrates 15 g	5%
Dietary fiber 3 g	12%
Sugars 3 g	
Protein 28 g	57%

Vitamin A 34%	•	Vitamin C 13%
Calcium 13%	•	Iron 18%
Vitamin E 10%	•	Folate 6%
Magnesium 7%	•	

* % Daily Values are based on a 2000 calorie diet.

© 2012 MenuTrinfo, LLC

Veggie Burger

Nutrition Facts

Serving size 10.6 oz

Amount per serving

Calories 330

Calories from fat 60

	% Daily Value *
Total fat 7 g	11%
Saturated fat 1.5 g	8%
Trans fat 0 g	
Sodium 650 mg	27%
Total carbohydrates 50 g	17%
Dietary fiber 11 g	46%
Sugars 10 g	
Protein 23 g	46%

Vitamin A 98%	•	Vitamin C 37%
Calcium 18%	•	Iron 22%
Vitamin E 25%	•	Folate 10%
Magnesium 5%	•	

* % Daily Values are based on a 2000 calorie diet.

© 2012 MenuTrinfo, LLC

Converting from a standard hamburger to a veggie burger opens up a world of tasty options. If you grill your veggie burger and top it with plenty of pickles, you'll never taste the difference.

Look at the differences in the calories from fat! There's almost three times the amount of fat in a cheeseburger compared to a veggie burger, and it's all the inflammatory saturated fat. There's also no cholesterol in the veggie burger. All that cancer-preventing dietary fiber is tripled, too. The protein content is virtually identical.

Hot Dog

Nutrition Facts
Serving size 2.7 oz

Amount per serving

Calories 170

   Calories from fat 90

                        % Daily Value *

Total fat 10 g	15%
Saturated fat 4.0 g	19%
Trans fat 0 g	
Cholesterol 15 mg	6%
Sodium 470 mg	20%
Total carbohydrates 15 g	5%
Sugars 4 g	
Protein 6 g	11%

Vitamin A 1%	●	Vitamin C 4%
Calcium 4%	●	Iron 7%
Vitamin E < 1%	●	Folate 8%
Magnesium 3%	●	

* % Daily Values are based on a 2000 calorie diet.

© 2012 MenuTrinfo, LLC

Vegetarian Hot Dog

Nutrition Facts
Serving size 4.7 oz

Amount per serving

Calories 190

   Calories from fat 30

                        % Daily Value *

Total fat 3.0 g	5%
Saturated fat 0.5 g	3%
Trans fat 0 g	
Sodium 780 mg	32%
Total carbohydrates 28 g	9%
Dietary fiber 3 g	13%
Sugars 8 g	
Protein 13 g	26%

Vitamin A 3%	●	Vitamin C 7%
Calcium 5%	●	Iron 10%
Vitamin E 1%	●	Folate 14%
Magnesium 6%	●	

* % Daily Values are based on a 2000 calorie diet.

© 2012 MenuTrinfo, LLC

A veggie hot dog has 1/8 the saturated fat of an ordinary hot dog. Calorie for calorie, veggie dogs have twice as much protein. There's no dietary fiber in an ordinary hot dog, either.

Chili Comparison

Nutrition Facts

Serving size 16.2 oz

Amount per serving

Calories 490

Calories from fat 190

	% Daily Value *
Total fat 22 g	34%
Saturated fat 8 g	40%
Trans fat 1.5 g	
Cholesterol 105 mg	34%
Sodium 1740 mg	73%
Total carbohydrates 33 g	11%
Dietary fiber 7 g	29%
Sugars 13 g	
Protein 37 g	75%

Vitamin A 24%	•	Vitamin C 33%
Calcium 12%	•	Iron 40%
Vitamin E 6%	•	Folate 15%
Magnesium 26%	•	

* % Daily Values are based on a 2000 calorie diet.

© 2012 MenuTrinfo, LLC

Granny's Slow Cooker Vegetarian Chili

Nutrition Facts

Serving size 23.5 oz

Amount per serving

Calories 470

Calories from fat 35

	% Daily Value *
Total fat 4.0 g	6%
Saturated fat 0.5 g	3%
Trans fat 0 g	
Sodium 1700 mg	71%
Total carbohydrates 96 g	32%
Dietary fiber 23 g	94%
Sugars 20 g	
Protein 23 g	46%

Vitamin A 35%	•	Vitamin C 198%
Calcium 22%	•	Iron 51%
Vitamin E 9%	•	Folate 59%
Magnesium 43%	•	

* % Daily Values are based on a 2000 calorie diet.

© 2012 MenuTrinfo, LLC

Look at the impressive differences in fat, cholesterol, fiber and Vitamin C. Just by taking the meat out of your chili, you triple your dietary fiber and increase your Vitamin C by over 500%

Meatloaf

Nutrition Facts

Serving size 10.7 oz

Amount per serving

Calories 510

Calories from fat 230

% Daily Value *

Total fat 26 g	41%
Saturated fat 10 g	50%
Trans fat 1.5 g	
Cholesterol 170 mg	56%
Sodium 1040 mg	43%
Total carbohydrates 29 g	10%
Sugars 24 g	
Protein 39 g	77%

Vitamin A 9%	Vitamin C 14%
Calcium 11%	Iron 24%
Vitamin E 4%	Folate 11%
Magnesium 12%	

* % Daily Values are based on a 2000 calorie diet.

© 2012 MenuTrinfo, LLC

Lighter Cajun Red Beans And Rice

Nutrition Facts

Serving size 25.8 oz

Amount per serving

Calories 530

Calories from fat 30

% Daily Value *

Total fat 3.0 g	5%
Saturated fat 0.5 g	4%
Trans fat 0 g	
Sodium 1300 mg	54%
Total carbohydrates 104 g	35%
Dietary fiber 26 g	102%
Sugars 15 g	
Protein 25 g	50%

Vitamin A 19%	Vitamin C 159%
Calcium 17%	Iron 40%
Vitamin E 5%	Folate 28%
Magnesium 49%	

* % Daily Values are based on a 2000 calorie diet.

© 2012 MenuTrinfo, LLC

Cut 23 grams of fat, add 26 grams of fiber, cut your sugar by almost half and triple your folate and magnesium without compromising your iron or your protein. And get a load of the serving size! You'll be eating for a really long time. Which is something I really like to do.

Pasta Comparison

Lasagna

Nutrition Facts

Serving size 11.5 oz

Amount per serving

Calories 560

Calories from fat 280

% Daily Value *

Total fat 32 g	49%
Saturated fat 14 g	69%
Trans fat 1.0 g	
Cholesterol 165 mg	54%
Sodium 1250 mg	52%
Total carbohydrates 22 g	7%
Dietary fiber 3 g	11%
Sugars 7 g	
Protein 46 g	91%

Vitamin A 18%	•	Vitamin C 16%	
Calcium 55%	•	Iron 26%	
Vitamin E 13%	•	Folate 9%	
Magnesium 13%	•		

* % Daily Values are based on a 2000 calorie diet.

© 2012 MenuTrinfo, LLC

Portabella Mushroom Pasta Toss

Nutrition Facts

Serving size 17.7 oz

Amount per serving

Calories 510

Calories from fat 130

% Daily Value *

Total fat 15 g	23%
Saturated fat 2.5 g	13%
Trans fat 0 g	
Cholesterol 4 mg	1%
Sodium 880 mg	36%
Total carbohydrates 83 g	28%
Dietary fiber 10 g	40%
Sugars 24 g	
Protein 14 g	29%

Vitamin A 32%	•	Vitamin C 12%	
Calcium 6%	•	Iron 23%	
Vitamin E 8%	•	Folate 15%	
Magnesium 12%	•		

* % Daily Values are based on a 2000 calorie diet.

© 2012 MenuTrinfo, LLC

In addition to adding a rich, meaty flavor to pasta dishes, some mushrooms are also a good source of Vitamin D. Look to mushrooms to cut the fat and increase the portion size without adding a lot of extra calories.

Mexican Chef Salad

Nutrition Facts

Serving size 15.5 oz

Amount per serving

Calories 910

Calories from fat 540

	% Daily Value *
Total fat 61 g	95%
Saturated fat 20 g	99%
Trans fat 0.5 g	
Cholesterol 130 mg	44%
Sodium 1080 mg	45%
Total carbohydrates 48 g	16%
Dietary fiber 10 g	42%
Sugars 7 g	
Protein 40 g	80%

Vitamin A 91%	•	Vitamin C 52%
Calcium 55%	•	Iron 31%
Vitamin E 35%	•	Folate 41%
Magnesium 32%	•	

* % Daily Values are based on a 2000 calorie diet.

© 2012 MenuTrinfo, LLC

Aztec Black Bean Salad

Nutrition Facts

Serving size 49.4 oz

Amount per serving

Calories 910

Calories from fat 70

	% Daily Value *
Total fat 8 g	12%
Saturated fat 1.0 g	6%
Trans fat 0 g	
Sodium 3520 mg	147%
Total carbohydrates 186 g	62%
Dietary fiber 46 g	183%
Sugars 26 g	
Protein 42 g	84%

Vitamin A 138%	•	Vitamin C 559%
Calcium 28%	•	Iron 90%
Vitamin E 29%	•	Folate 143%
Magnesium 75%	•	

* % Daily Values are based on a 2000 calorie diet.

© 2012 MenuTrinfo, LLC

The serving size here is unrealistic, but that's the point. Filling up on vegetables will fill you up without making you fat. The micronutrient content of a great salad is mind-blowing. Eat a salad every day as your preferred lunch selection.

Sandwich Comparison

Crusty Grilled Ham And Cheese Sandwiches

Nutrition Facts

Serving size 3.2 oz

Amount per serving

Calories 230

   Calories from fat 100

	% Daily Value *
Total fat 11 g	17%
Saturated fat 6 g	31%
Trans fat 0 g	
Cholesterol 35 mg	12%
Sodium 630 mg	26%
Total carbohydrates 20 g	7%
Dietary fiber 1 g	4%
Protein 11 g	23%

Vitamin A 7%	•	Vitamin C 4%
Calcium 17%	•	Iron 9%
Vitamin E 7%	•	Folate 2%
Magnesium 3%	•	

* % Daily Values are based on a 2000 calorie diet.

© 2012 MenuTrinfo, LLC

English Muffin, Hummus, & Tomato Sandwich

Nutrition Facts

Serving size 3.4 oz

Amount per serving

Calories 190

   Calories from fat 25

	% Daily Value *
Total fat 2.5 g	4%
Saturated fat 0 g	2%
Trans fat 0 g	
Sodium 570 mg	24%
Total carbohydrates 34 g	11%
Dietary fiber 3 g	13%
Sugars 1 g	
Protein 7 g	15%

Vitamin A 3%	•	Vitamin C 4%
Calcium 14%	•	Iron 14%
Vitamin E 1%	•	Folate 14%
Magnesium 11%	•	

* % Daily Values are based on a 2000 calorie diet.

© 2012 MenuTrinfo, LLC

Making a grilled sandwich on a weekend or at lunchtime can be a real dietary disaster. Switching to a similar sized sandwich made with toast and hummus with a slice of tomato is a tasty, satisfying alternative that doesn't make a mess of your stovetop.

Zesty Chicken Stir-fry

Nutrition Facts

Serving size 16.0 oz

Amount per serving

Calories 540

   Calories from fat 130

	% Daily Value *
Total fat 15 g	23%
Saturated fat 3.0 g	14%
Trans fat 0 g	
Cholesterol 130 mg	43%
Sodium 2030 mg	85%
Total carbohydrates 47 g	16%
Dietary fiber 10 g	39%
Sugars 21 g	
Protein 56 g	111%

Vitamin A 182%	•	Vitamin C 17%
Calcium 9%	•	Iron 22%
Vitamin E 46%	•	Folate 13%
Magnesium 26%	•	

* % Daily Values are based on a 2000 calorie diet.

© 2012 MenuTrinfo, LLC

Veggie Tofu Stir-fry with Sesame Seeds Over Brown R

Nutrition Facts

Serving size 25.5 oz

Amount per serving

Calories 570

   Calories from fat 260

	% Daily Value *
Total fat 29 g	45%
Saturated fat 4.0 g	20%
Trans fat 0 g	
Sodium 1010 mg	42%
Total carbohydrates 45 g	15%
Dietary fiber 14 g	55%
Sugars 9 g	
Protein 45 g	91%

Vitamin A 65%	•	Vitamin C 304%
Calcium 172%	•	Iron 55%
Vitamin E 13%	•	Folate 49%
Magnesium 57%	•	

* % Daily Values are based on a 2000 calorie diet.

© 2012 MenuTrinfo, LLC

Why not skip the chicken in your stir-fry, and opt for brown rice instead? All the yummy seasoning comes from the added spices, and not the meat itself. I prepare a stir fry at least once a week for Ice Daughter and me to enjoy at home.

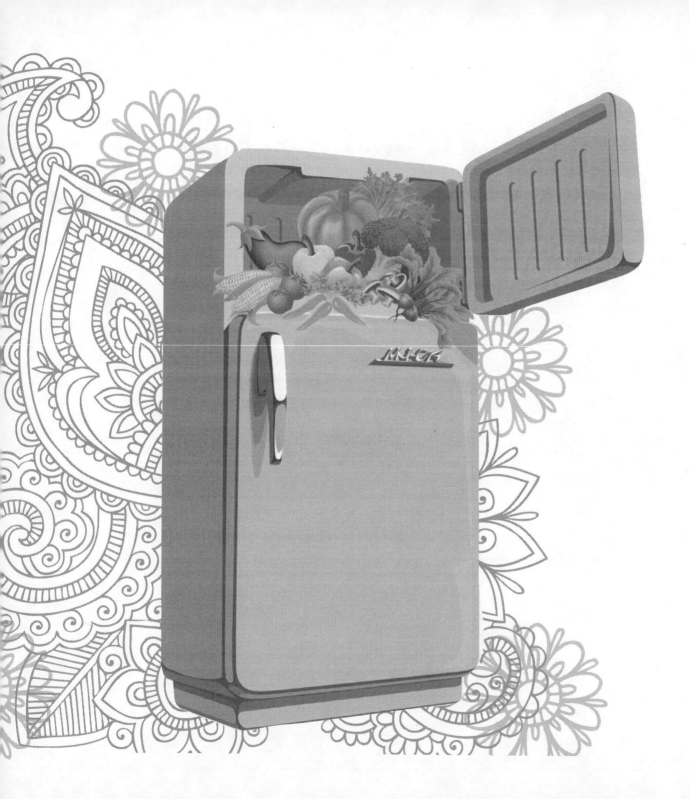

Recipes for You
— Dr. Mary —

My fridge looks a little different than it used to. The outside looks the same, of course, but now the cheese tray is full of tofu and soy sausage. The milk jug is replaced with soy milk. We always have a re-sealable container of rinsed, drained beans, some prepared grain, a loaf of great bread and hummus, all of which replaced the yogurt and string cheese. I think you'll enjoy some of my favorite recipes, made with foods I love in my little kitchen. You'll also enjoy a nice collection of recipes contributed by vegan chefs and excellent local restaurants.

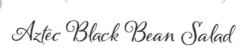

Aztec Black Bean Salad

Ingredients

2 (15 oz.) cans black beans, drained and rinsed
1/2 cup finely chopped red onions
1 green bell pepper, seeded and diced
1 red bell pepper, seeded and diced
1 (15 oz.) can corn kernels, drained, or 1 (10 oz) bag frozen corn
2-3 tomatoes, diced
3/4 cup chopped cilantro (optional)
3 teaspoons seasoned rice vinegar
2 tablespoons apple or distilled vinegar
Juice of 1 lemon or 1 lime
2 garlic cloves, finely minced
2 teaspoon ground cumin
1 teaspoon coriander
1/2 teaspoon red pepper flakes or 1 pinch cayenne
1 chipotle chili, canned in adobe sauce, diced

Directions

In a large bowl, combine beans, onion, bell peppers, corn, tomatoes and cilantro. Whisk together vinegars, lemon juice, garlic, cumin, coriander, red pepper flakes and chipotle. Pour over salad and toss. Serve immediately.

~ Dr. Mary

Granny's Slow Cooker Vegetarian Chili

Ingredients

1 (11 oz.) can condensed black bean soup (or canned black beans in juice)
1 (15 oz.) can kidney beans, drained and rinsed
1 (15 oz.) can garbanzo beans, drained and rinsed
1 (16 oz.) can vegetarian baked beans
1 (29 oz.) can crushed tomatoes
1 (15 oz.) can whole kernel corn, drained
1 onion, chopped
1 green bell pepper, chopped
2 zucchini, chopped
2 stalks celery, chopped
2 garlic cloves, chopped
1 (4 oz.) can diced chilies
1-2 jalapenos, chopped
1 tablespoon chili powder
2 teaspoons cumin
1 tablespoon dried parsley
1 teaspoon dried oregano
1 tablespoon dried basil
1 tablespoon cilantro (optional)

Directions

In a saucepan, saute the onion, bell pepper, zucchini and celery for 5 minutes. In a slow cooker, combine black bean soup, kidney beans, garbanzo beans, baked beans, tomatoes, corn, onion, bell pepper, zucchini, jalapeno, chilies and celery. Add garlic, chili powder, cumin, parsley, oregano, basil and cilantro

Cook for about 6 hours on low.

Serve with tortillas or cornbread.

~ Dr. Mary

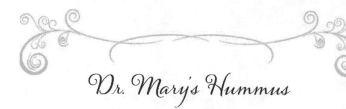

Dr. Mary's Hummus

1 ginormous (29 oz.) can garbanzo beans
1/3 cup tahini (this is just crushed sesame seeds)
8 drops of Tabasco sauce
Salt and pepper to taste
1 garlic clove, crushed

Rinse well and drain the garbanzo beans. Throw all the ingredients into the food processor and whiz until combined. You may need to add up to 1/4 cup of water and scrape the sides a few times. Serve with raw veggies or baked tortillas cut into wedges.

~ Dr. Mary

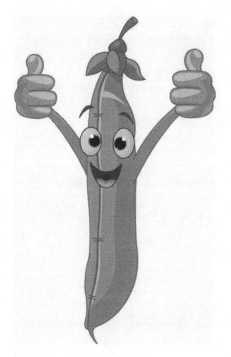

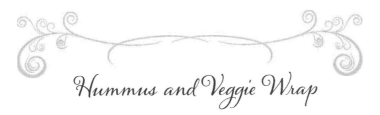

Hummus and Veggie Wrap

Ingredients

1 12-inch whole grain or spelt tortilla
1/2 cup hummus
1/8 cup cucumbers
1/8 cup diced tomatoes
1/8 cup bell peppers
1/8 cup shoestring carrots
3 slices red onions
Alfalfa sprouts
Lettuce

Directions

Warm tortilla for a few minutes in a frypan on low to soften. Spread the hummus over the tortilla, add assorted veggies, saving the lettuce for last. Roll up, tucking in the edges. Slice in half or eat whole.

Add a touch of hot sauce if you like.

~ Dr. Mary

Lighter Cajun Red Beans and Rice

Ingredients

1 large onion, chopped
2 garlic cloves
30 oz. canned red kidney beans, rinsed and drained
8 oz. low sodium tomato sauce
2 green or red bell peppers, chopped
1 teaspoon dried oregano
1 teaspoon dried thyme
1 teaspoon hot pepper sauce
2 cups brown rice
1/3 cup fresh chives or chopped scallions, for garnish

Directions

Cook the rice according to the package directions. Meanwhile, coat a large nonstick skillet with nonstick spray, and warm over medium-high heat. You can also just use a little water. Add onion and garlic and cook, stirring for 5 minutes, or until tender.

Stir in the beans, tomato sauce, bell peppers, oregano, thyme, and hot pepper sauce. Simmer for 15 minutes.

Serve the beans over the rice.

~ Dr. Mar

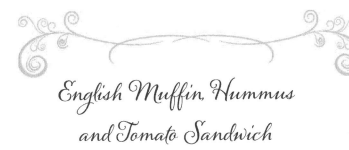

English Muffin, Hummus and Tomato Sandwich

Ingredients

1 multi-grain English muffin
1 tomato, sliced
1 tablespoon hummus
Salt & pepper, to taste

Directions

Toast the English muffin halves. Spread the hummus on each half and leave open-face.

Place tomato slices on top of the hummus. Sprinkle with salt and pepper. We eat this sandwich frequently, using different breads and pickled vegetables to enhance the flavor.

~ Dr. Mary

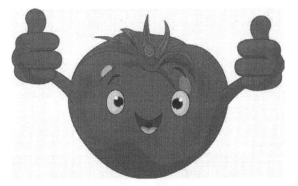

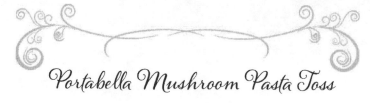

Portabella Mushroom Pasta Toss

Ingredients

1 red onion
2 garlic cloves chopped
2 tablespoons olive oil (or just substitute water)
5 portabella mushroom caps, scrubbed and sliced into strips or diced
Fresh basil, snipped, to taste
1 (26 oz.) jars marinara sauce (cheeseless)
16 oz. box of whole wheat pasta, any shape

Directions

In a large pot, bring 5 quarts of water to a boil. Add the pasta (and salt if desired) and cook for 8-12 minutes.

In a second large pot, heat olive oil. Add red onion and stir until lightly caramelized. Add garlic and cook for one minute, being careful not to burn it. Add the mushrooms and cook until they are cooked down and softened. Add marinara and basil. Cook for 10 minutes.

When pasta finishes cooking, drain well, reserving a few tablespoons of the pasta water. Add pasta and small amount of pasta water to sauce.

Garnish with coarsely chopped fresh basil.

~ Dr. Mary

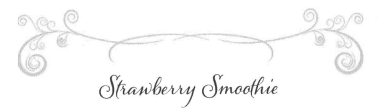

Strawberry Smoothie

Ingredients

(Makes 2 1-cup servings)

1 cup frozen strawberries
1 medium frozen banana
1/2 - 1 cup vanilla rice milk

Directions

Place all ingredients in a blender. Blend at high speed until smooth.

~ Dr. Mary

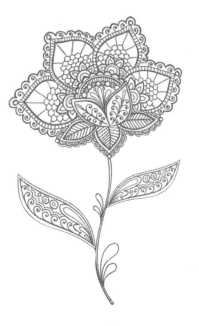

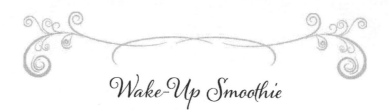

Wake-Up Smoothie

I like to drink one of these about an hour before a run. Gives me TONS of energy and puts my calcium anxiety at rest. Feel free to use whatever you have in your refrigerator.

~ *Anne Stanton*

2 handfuls of blueberries
1 banana or a soft peach
2 tablespoons of nut butter
1 tablespoon of honey
1 ½ cups of almond milk (fortified with calcium!)
¼ teaspoon salt
A couple of handfuls of kale or spinach
5 or 6 ice cubes

Put the ingredients in a blender and whir away!

Inspiration came from nomeatathlete.com, my favorite website. Lots of great recipes and exercise advice!

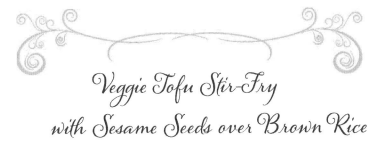

Veggie Tofu Stir-Fry
with Sesame Seeds over Brown Rice

Ingredients

2 lbs firm tofu, cut into 1-inch cubes
3 tablespoon soy sauce
2 1/4 cups vegetable broth or water
3/4 cup brown rice
1 tablespoon canola oil or olive oil (or just use water)
4 cloves garlic, minced
1 medium yellow onions, thinly sliced
1 lb broccoli, cut into pieces

2 large red peppers, cored, seeded and thinly sliced
1/2 lb button mushrooms, thinly sliced
1 (6 oz) can water chestnuts, drained
1/2 teaspoon dried basil
1/2 teaspoon dried oregano
1/2 teaspoon ground black pepper
1/4 cup sesame seeds

Directions

Place tofu in a colander and drain 10 minutes, then pat dry with paper towels.

Place soy sauce in a shallow dish, add tofu, cover, refrigerate and marinate 15 minutes or up to 1 hour.

In medium covered saucepan, bring 2 cups vegetable broth or water to a boil. Slowly stir in rice, cover and reduce heat to low. Simmer 40 minutes, or until all the water is absorbed.

Meanwhile, heat the oil in a wok, large skillet, or heavy saucepan over medium-high heat. Add garlic and onion and saute 1-2 minutes.

Add broccoli and red peppers, the remaining 1 1/4 cup broth or water, and cook, stirring frequently for about 5 minutes. Add mushrooms, water chestnuts, basil, oregano, and black pepper and continue to cook 2 more minutes.

Add sesame seeds and the marinated tofu with soy sauce, and cook, stirring gently, about 5 minutes.

Serve over the cooked rice.

~ Dr. Mary

Zucchini Chocolate Chip Vegan Cookies

1 cup Earth Balance margarine, softened
2 cups granulated sugar
2 egg equivalent of Ener-G Egg Replacer
4 cups all-purpose flour
2 teaspoons baking soda
2 teaspoons ground cinnamon
1 teaspoon salt
2 small zucchini, grated (approximately 2 cups of grated zucchini)
2 cups semi-sweet chocolate chips
2 cups walnuts, chopped (optional)

Preheat oven to 350 degrees. Spray cookie sheets with cooking spray or lightly oil. Next cream margarine and sugar together in a large mixing bowl until fluffy. Then add the Egg Replacer and dry ingredients. Mix well.

Stir in the zucchini. When well mixed, fill in walnuts and chocolate chips. Drop by teaspoonfuls with two inches between each cookie onto the cookie sheet. Let stand to cool for 2 to 3 minutes, then remove from the cookie sheet and cool completely.

~ Dr. Mary (adapted from love4culinary)

Ice Daughter loves to make these. She found the recipe on the food.com website (love4culinary) and switched out the animal-based ingredients for plant-based ones. They are amazingly yummy, but don't be fooled. Just because they're vegan, doesn't mean they're not fattening. These really are, but if you're going to indulge occasionally, your dessert should taste this good.

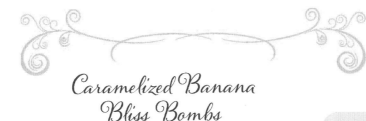

Caramelized Banana Bliss Bombs

Who would be interested in a dessert that is all at once healthy, elegant, easy, quick, and downright scrumptious?
Me. And hopefully you!

Caramelized Banana Bliss Bombs is one of my favorite desserts—the recipe is easy to make, healthy, and really scrumptious. I hope you love it too!

Spiced Sauce:

One 12.3 oz. container of silken tofu (firm)
½ cup pure maple syrup
2 tablespoons oil (sunflower, melted coconut, non-virgin olive, or safflower)
¼ teaspoon each: ground cardamom and ground cinnamon
⅛ teaspoon sea salt

Flair:

1½ cups sliced strawberries
2 tablespoons crushed or chopped pecans (raw or dry toasted)

~ Radiant Health, Inner Wealth

MEET THE TALENTED CHEF TESS CHALLIS!

Ice Daughter and I were invited to a vegan cooking class with author and vegan chef Tess Challis. It was a sunny, warm Sunday evening, and we were bicycling to the event, when I started wondering if we could have more fun just staying on our bikes and zipping around downtown, maybe even heading to the bay for a quick swim.

Lucky me! Instead of just another swim in the big pond, I got to learn a great new way to prepare and save whole foods.

Tess taught us how to make delish soda style drinks out of ginger and lime with our Soda Stream*, which I never thought of. She made some yummy baked zucchini with a crispy polenta crust. Then she blew my mind by popping amaranth. I had no idea that any food could be popped besides popcorn. Check out Tess' seriously cool cookbooks at www.radianthealth-innerwealth.com. We bought all three, and plan to cook through all three, and then we are going to attend every single cooking class she presents, until Tess and I are both little old vegan ladies together, chasing Ice Daughter's great grandkids around.

*A carbonator that costs about $100. In addition to carbonating water, you can add flavorings to make your own soda.

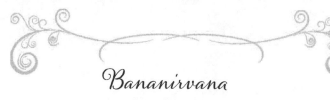

Bananirvana

3 firm bananas (not overly ripe)
1 tablespoon sucanat or packed brown sugar
1 teaspoon vanilla powder (optional but delicious!)*
1 tablespoon non-hydrogenated margarine

In a blender, combine the tofu, maple syrup, oil, cardamom, cinnamon, and salt until very smooth and consistently creamy. Set aside (or refrigerate for up to a week).

Prepare the strawberries and pecans and set them aside.

Slice each banana in half lengthwise. Next, slice each banana half in half width-wise so that you end up with twelve banana segments that are each half of their original thickness and length.

Mix the sucanat and vanilla and lightly coat each banana segment evenly with the mixture. Alternately, you can throw caution to the wind and simply sprinkle the sugar and vanilla on each piece of banana.

Heat a very large skillet over medium-high heat. Add the margarine. When the margarine is melted, distribute it evenly over the pan.

Place the banana pieces in a single layer on the pan. Allow them to get nicely browned on the bottom (this should take well under 5 minutes). Gently flip them over with a heat proof spatula and allow them to brown on the other side. When both sides are gloriously browned and caramelized, turn off the heat.

To serve: Place the desired amount of sauce on a dessert plate. Top with three of the banana segments and garnish with some strawberries and pecans. Repeat for the remaining three portions. Serve immediately if you know what's good for you.

Serves 4; 30 minutes or under!

~ Tess Challis

Hungarian Chickpeas!

Holy bean love, people...these are insanely delicious! They're very quick and easy to put together, but do require smoked paprika. You can usually find this divine elixir of spice in health food stores, many supermarkets and most international food markets. It's worth the (relatively inexpensive) purchase though. Smoked paprika will lend a rich, earthy, complex flavor like nothing else. It's also great sprinkled on baba ganoush or hummus, or as a seasoning for a wide variety of dishes. Welcome to my new obsession.

15 oz. can chickpeas (garbanzo beans), rinsed and drained
2 tablespoons pitted and quartered kalamata olives (or other Greek olives)
2 tablespoons each: raisins, chopped cilantro, and minced yellow or white onion
1 tablespoon each: extra-virgin olive oil and raw agave nectar
2 teaspoons each: Dijon mustard, fresh lime juice, and smoked paprika
1 teaspoon dried oregano
2 large cloves garlic, minced or pressed
½ teaspoon sea salt

Combine all of the ingredients and stir very well. Serve cold or at room temperature. This will keep, refrigerated in an airtight container, for up to a week.

~ Radiance 4 Life

Oven Roasted Cauliflower with Rosemary and Garlic

Here's the perfect solution for when you have the munchies, but want to give your body something healthy! This dish is so yummy that I've been known, in moments I'm not proud of, to eat an entire batch of this at one time! Don't be like me...share the goodness. Incidentally, this is a great side dish for Thanksgiving (or any special occasion) and can be prepared in advance. Simply toss all of the ingredients together and marinate overnight. Pop it into the oven half an hour before dinner, and there go you! Simple elegance.

2 teaspoons fresh rosemary leaf, stems removed and chopped
4 teaspoons olive oil, extra-virgin or regular
6 medium cloves garlic, minced or pressed
½ teaspoon sea salt (plus up to ⅛ teaspoon more if you like)
¼ teaspoon each: organic sugar (or sucanat) and ground black pepper
½ teaspoon balsamic vinegar
3½ cups chopped cauliflower (cut into bite sized pieces)

1. Preheat the oven to 400° F. Place everything but the cauliflower in a large bowl and stir to mix. Next, add the cauliflower and combine well with the seasonings using a rubber spatula. At this point you can allow the mixture to marinate for up to 24 hours (refrigerated in an airtight container) if you like.

2. Spread the mixture onto a large ungreased cookie sheet, using the rubber spatula to scrape all of the herbs and spices onto the cauliflower. Bake for about 15 minutes.

3. Turn the cauliflower over with a heat proof spatula and bake for another 10-15 minutes, or until lightly browned and very tender. Remove and serve. Feel impressed with yourself for as long as you like.

Serves 2; 30 minutes or under!

~ Radiant Health, Inner Wealth

128

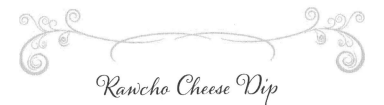

Rawcho Cheese Dip

This dip is my latest obsession——I even dream about it. (You've been warned.) And it stars one of THE stars of the plant-based (vegan) kingdom - cashews. From creamy sauces to smooth dips to raw key lime pies, cashews are perfect in a huge variety of dishes. Plus they're nutrient-dense as well, which makes them 100% pure awesome!

½ cup raw cashews
4 oz. jar pimientos, drained
¼cup nutritional yeast powder
3 tablespoons fresh lemon juice
3 medium-large cloves garlic, peeled
2 tablespoons water
1 teaspoon granulated onion
¾ teaspoon sea salt
¼ teaspoon ground cayenne

Blend all of the ingredients in a food processor (or good blender) until completely smooth. Serve cold or at room temperature with raw vegetables, baked tortilla chips, or raw crackers. This will store, refrigerated in an airtight container, for at least a week.

Makes about 1 cup of dip (4 servings)
30 Minutes or Under!

~ Radiant 4 Life

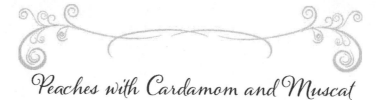

Peaches with Cardamom and Muscat

1 bottle Muscat wine
1 vanilla bean, halved with the seeds scraped out
6 cardamom pods, ground -- about one teaspoon
4 ripe, unblemished peaches

Combine the wine, vanilla bean and cardamom in a pot and bring to a boil. Lower heat to a simmer and cook for 5 minutes. Add the peaches and poach for 15 minutes more. Take the peaches out, turn the heat up to a boil and reduce until about 1 cup of liquid remains. We like this served warm, but it's also delicious cold the next day. To plate, cut the peaches in half, removing the peels and the pits. Arrange two of the peach halves in a bowl and pour on some of the sauce.

~ Cooks' House: The Art and Soul
of Sustainable Cuisine

WELCOME TO THE FABULOUS COOKS' HOUSE!

When I was studying for my upcoming internal medicine board recertification, I dined frequently at the Cooks' House, a tiny restaurant with giganto flavors. My go-to order was an exquisitely flavored potatoes and greens dish. I'd look over my plate at Ice Daughter and think how lucky we were to be eating such incredible food together.

The Cooks' House is not a vegan restaurant, but the two chefs never made a fuss about accommodating my requests. I didn't have to call ahead at the Cooks' House, but I do know some chefs do appeciate an advance head's up.

I love what chefs Eric Patterson and Jennifer Blakeslee wrote in their cookbook, *Cooks' House: The Art and Soul of Sustainable Cuisine*, from which these recipes are taken.

"When it comes to top notch-ingredients, Michigan will give you a run for the money to anywhere else on earth. We have small farmers who lovingly grow the highest quality produce. Depending on the time of year, we get morels, golden chanterelles, porcinis, hen of the woods, hunter's hearts and other wild mushrooms foraged by the area's foremost expert. There are wild leeks, wild watercress, wild roses, wild fennel—all of which we use when we can get them.

Marco Pierre White is fond of saying that Mother Nature is the true artist. We take his advice in this matter, choosing to let the ingredients speak for themselves while keeping our dishes as simple as possible. With all the world-class products we have to work with, keeping the dishes simple is only too easy."

Apricots Poached with Ginger and Lime

1/2 cup sugar
1/2 cup Riesling
A piece of ginger about the size of a wine cork, cut in half lengthwise, then each half cut into 6 pieces
1 vanilla bean, split in half with the beans scraped out
12 firm, ripe apricots
Zest of 2 limes

Mix the sugar, wine and 1/2 cup water in a pot and bring to a boil. Stir well until the sugar dissolves. Add the ginger and the vanilla. Simmer for 5 minutes. Add the apricots and simmer 2 more minutes. Remove from the heat, add the zest and allow to cool. When the mixture has cooled, remove the apricots. Cut them in half and discard the pits. Put the apricots back into the sauce. To serve, divide the apricots into bowls and spoon over some of the sauce.

~ Cooks' House: The Art and Soul
   of Sustainable Cuisine

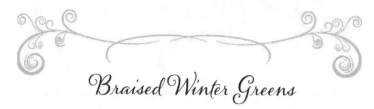

Braised Winter Greens

1 tablespoon olive oil
1/2 onion, sliced with the grain
2 cloves garlic, peeled and sliced
3 stalks Swiss chard, cut into 2-inch pieces, stems discarded
3 stalks green kale, cut into 2-inch pieces, stems discarded
1 cup vegetable stock

Put the olive oil into a 2-quart pan along with the onion and garlic. Season with salt and pepper. Add the greens and saute for about 3 minutes over medium heat or until they are wilted. Add the vegetable stock and continue to cook for 4 minutes more. Adjust the seasoning. Serve in its own bowl.

*~ Cook's House: The Art and Soul
of Sustainable Cuisine*

Warm Indian Creamed Rice with Pomegranates and Pistachios

1 quart soy milk
1/3 cup short grain rice
1 inch piece of whole cinnamon
1 clove
3 cardamom seeds, gently ground; don't make a powder out of it
6 tablespoons sugar
1/2 cup pomegranate seeds
1/2 cup pistachios
2 tablespoons orange juice

Bring the milk to a boil in a 2-quart pot. Remove it from the heat, dip out 1/2 cup of the liquid and reserve. Give the rice a good washing in a colander and add it to the milk still in the pot. Put the milk and rice mixture back on low heat and cook, stirring, for 20 minutes. Add the cinnamon stick, clove and cardamom. Cover the pot and continue to cook on low heat for 1 hour, stirring the rice every 15 minutes.

Wait, we're not done: add the sugar and the pomegranates and cook for another hour. At this point you'll need to keep a close eye on the pot. Continue stirring every 15 minutes. If it starts to get too thick or stick to the pan, add a splash more milk from the reserve. When the second hour is finished, remove the cinnamon stick and the clove. Stir in the pistachios and orange juice. Now, spoon the rick mixture into four bowls and let it cool down completely. We personally don't like this chilled. Give it a taste and choose what suites you.

~ Cooks' House: The Art and Soul
of Sustainable Cuisine

Roasted Red Pepper and Asparagus Crostini

1 whole garlic bulb
1 rosemary sprig
2 red bell peppers
Fustini's Tuscan Herb Extra Virgin Olive Oil
Salt and pepper to taste
1 French baguette
24 asparagus tips (reserve stalks for another use)
2 teaspoons Fustini's 18 Year Traditional Balsamic, plus more for drizzling

Preheat oven to 400 degrees.

Slice top off whole garlic bulb. Place bulb on a square of foil. Roast with a drizzle of Fustini's Tuscan Herb Extra Virgin Olive Oil, a pinch of salt, a grind of pepper and one rosemary sprig. Wrap foil around bulb. Cut peppers in half; remove ribs and seeds. Place on a sheet of foil or baking sheet. Brush with Fustini's Tuscan Herb Extra Virgin Olive Oil. Roast the garlic bulb and pepper halves 25-30 minutes or until garlic is soft and peppers begin to char. Set aside to cool.

Lower oven temperature to 350 degrees. To make crostini, slice baguette into 3/4-inch slices. Place on ungreased baking sheet. Toast 15 minutes or until golden. Meanwhile, in a large skillet, bring about 1/2 inch of water and salt to a boil. Add asparagus, reduce heat to a simmer, and cook for 3-5 minutes or until bright green and still somewhat resistant when pierced with the tip of a sharp knife; drain and cool.

Squeeze roasted garlic from bulbs into a small bowl; spread on crostini. Slice roasted red pepper into thin strips; place in a small bowl. Drizzle with 2 teaspoons Fustini's 18 Year Traditional Balsamic. Mix gently until peppers are coated. Place a few peppers on crostini and top with 2 steamed asparagus tips. Drizzle with a little Fustini's 18 Year Traditional Balsamic. Season to taste with salt and pepper.

~ In the Kitchen with Fustini's

YOU'LL LOVE WHAT'S COOKING AT FUSTINI'S!

In Italy, "Fustini" are the stainless steel containers in which olive oils and vinegars are stored. The word inspired the store name of my favorite specialty shop in all the land—a shop that sells extra virgin olive oil and balsamic vinegar, and pretty much only that. On the surface, it seems like a crazy idea. But owner Jim Milligan said the idea makes perfect sense in context of what has been happening in the food world in recent years: the quest for quality, the trend toward buying seasonal products from local vendors (olive oil is, in fact, a seasonal product), increasing numbers of health-conscious consumers and a renewed interest in home cooking. Today, people around the globe have fallen in love with balsamic vinegar and olive oil. The enterprise has been immensely successful, and three more locations have opened up around Michigan!

The recipes on this page are taken from *In the Kitchen with Fustini's*, a collection of recipes that will make your taste buds sing. They range from the simple to the sublime and feature familiar ingredients as well as some that may be new to you. I think you'll love the exciting new flavor combinations, which add a whole new dimension to plant-based eating.

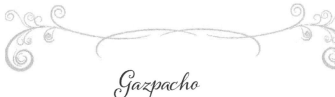

Gazpacho

1 tablespoon Fustini's Sherry Reserva Vinegar
1/8 cup Fustini's Manzanillo Extra Virgin Olive Oil
1-1/2-2 pounds large, ripe, flavorful tomatoes, chopped
1 medium Spanish onion, diced
2 garlic cloves, minced
1 red and 1 green bell pepper, dice (reserve 1 tablespoon each for garnish)
1 hothouse cucumber, seeded and diced (reserve 1 tablespoon for garnish)
1 thick slice day-old crusty white bread, softened in water
1 jalapeno pepper, ribs removed, seeded and minced
1 small bunch cilantro, 4 sprigs reserved for garnish, rest roughly chopped
Salt and pepper to taste
4 green onions, light green and white parts only, thinly sliced, for garnish

Place all ingredients up to and including cilantro in a blender or food processor and pulse until fairly smooth. Season to taste with salt and pepper. Chill at least 1 hour or overnight.

To serve, put an ice cube in a chilled bowl, pour cold soup over and garnish with diced pepper, cucumbers, green onions and cilantro sprig.

~ In the Kitchen with Fustini's

Curried Lentil Soup

1 pound brown or green lentils
2 tablespoons Fustini's Cilantro and Onion Extra Virgin Olive Oil
1 medium onion, chopped
3 carrots, chopped and sliced
2 stalks celery, chopped or sliced
2 large garlic cloves, pressed or finely chopped
1 teaspoon ground cumin, or to taste
2-4 tablespoons curry powder, or to taste
1 teaspoon chili garlic paste (optional)
1 bay leaf (remove after cooking)
1 14 1/2-ounce can diced or coarsely cut tomatoes with juice
3 cups fresh baby spinach leaves
2-3 quarts vegetable broth, divided
1 teaspoon fresh thyme leaves, chopped
2 teaspoons Fustini's 12 Year White Balsamic Vinegar
Salt and pepper to taste
Fresh flat-leaf parsley, chopped, for garnish

Rinse and pick through lentils. Set aside.

Saute onion, carrots and celery over medium heat in Fustini's Cilantro and Onion Extra Virgin Olive Oil. Add garlic, cumin, curry powder, chili-garlic paste (if using) and bay leaf and cook 1-2 minutes, or until fragrant.

Stir in tomatoes, spinach, and 2 cartons of veggie broth and bring to a boil. Add lentils and thyme, return to boil, then lower heat and simmer 35-40 minutes, or until lentils are softened but still hold their shape. Check during cooking and add more broth as needed to achieve desired consistency. Toward end of cooking time, add Fustini's 12 Year White Balsamic and stir.

Season to taste with salt and pepper. Garnish with a sprinkle of parsley.

~ In the Kitchen with Fustini's

Spaghetti Squash with Pomodoro Sauce

1 spaghetti squash (about 1 1/2 pounds)
2 garlic cloves, minced
1 small onion, finely chopped
1 teaspoon Fustini's Garlic Extra Virgin Olive Oil
1 teaspoon Fustini's Persian Lime Extra Virgin Olive Oil
3 tablespoons tomato paste
1/2 pound fresh plum tomatoes, roughly chopped
1 teaspoon Fustini's Champagne Vinegar
1 teaspoon dried oregano
1 teaspoon dried basil
1/2 teaspoon red pepper flakes
Fresh basil for garnish

Preheat oven to 375 degrees.

Halve squash lengthwise and scoop out the seeds. Coat a baking sheet with cooking spray; lay squash halves, flesh side down, on sheet. Bake 35 minutes or until shell can be easily pierced.

While squash bakes, saute garlic and onion in Fustini's Garlic Extra Virgin Olive Oil and Fustini's Persian Lime Extra Virgin Olive Oil over medium heat 5 minutes. Add remaining ingredients (except fresh basil) and cook, stirring occasionally, 30 minutes, Lower heat if sauce begins to boil.

Remove squash from oven. Scrape crosswise to pull strands from shell. Place squash in nonmetal serving bowl. Pour sauce over and garnish with fresh basil.

You can also cook the squash whole, halving and scooping the seeds out after cooking.

~ In the Kitchen with Fustini's

Chef A.J.'s "Hail to Kale" Salad

Even people who say that don't like kale will gobble this up. It's so delicious I often have two large bowls of it for breakfast!

Salad
2 large heads of curly kale (about 24 ounces)
chopped almonds

Dressing
1 cup raw almond butter (unsweetened and unsalted)
1 cup coconut water (or regular water)
¼ cup fresh lime juice (about 2) and zest
2 cloves garlic
Fresh peeled ginger (approximately 1" or ¾ of an ounce)
2 tablespoons low sodium Tamari
4 pitted dates (soaked in water if not soft)
½ teaspoon red pepper flakes

In a high-powered blender, combine all ingredients until smooth and creamy. Remove the thick, larger stems from the kale and place in a large bowl. Pour 2 cups of the dressing over the kale and using an Ulu blade, massage the dressing into the kale while using the Ulu to finely chop the kale. Sprinkle with seeds or nuts before serving, if desired.

Like a woman, this only gets better with age. This dressing also makes a delicious dip for fresh veggies but you need to cut way back on the water and add some cilantro. It's also delicious when made with peanut butter and you throw some shredded raw beets and carrots into the salad.

~ Chef A.J.

MEET THE INCREDIBLE CHEF A.J.!

If you are looking for inspiration, look to Chef A.J. She's dynamic and funny, and when I've felt like a task before me is insurmountable, she's the gal the makes me believe that anything is possible. She is inspiring, energetic and committed to her vegan lifestyle. Enjoy her recipes and a very personal biography in her book, *Unprocessed*.

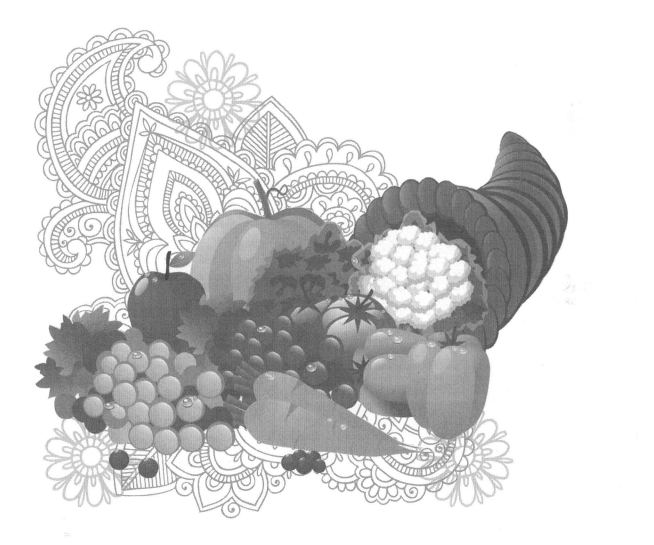

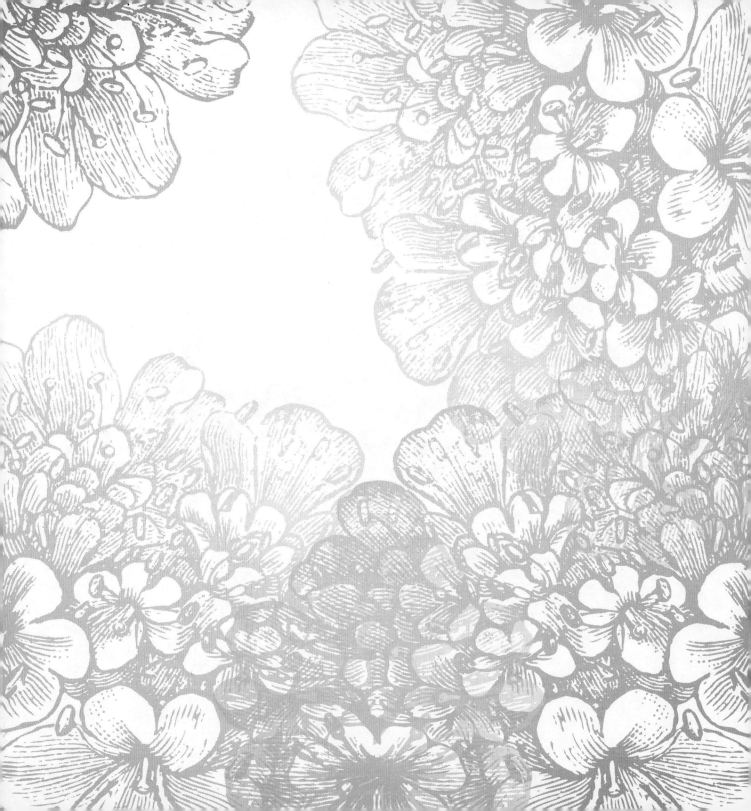

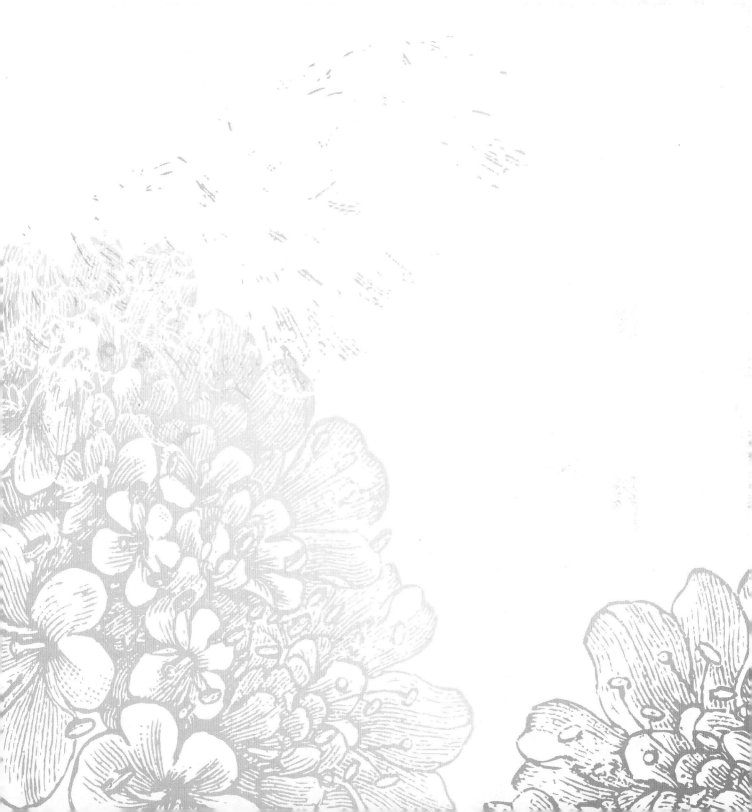

Made in the USA
San Bernardino, CA
14 February 2013